Decoding the

Enigma

Decoding the

Enigma

The real reasons for the decline
of our country

Understanding our
declining national character
and its relationship to
degenerative diseases
like Alzheimer's
and depression

MaryAlice E. Bonwell

Printed in the United States of America

ISBN: 978-0-9889511-4-3 trade paperback
ISBN: 978-0-9889511-5-0 e-book

Drawings by Jim Mathenia

DEDICATION

Weston A. Price, D.D.S.
Nutrition and Physical Degeneration

Francis M. Pottenger, Jr., M.D.
Pottenger's Cats

Theron G. Randolph, M.D.
An Alternative Approach to Allergies

Doris J. Rapp, M.D.
Is This Your Child?
Is This Your Child's World?
Our Toxic World

William J. Rea, M.D.
Volume I Chemical Sensitivity: Principles
and Mechanisms
Volume II Sources of Total Body Load
Volume III Clinical Manifestations of
Pollutant Overload
Volume IV Tools of Diagnosis and Methods
of Treatment

ACKNOWLEDGMENTS

Pat Connolly, former executive director of the Price-Pottenger Nutrition Foundation, was the first to urge me to combine my experience as a special education teacher with my interest in the works of Drs. Price and Pottenger. She was known for her willingness to mentor others. Her encouragement and enthusiasm were and will always be important to me. I want to thank the PPNF for allowing me to quote from their materials and for the role that they have played in preserving the works of Weston A. Price, D.D.S., Francis M. Pottenger, Jr., MD., and other nutritional pioneers.

I also want to express my deep gratitude to my two wonderful, dedicated, competent teacher aides, Irene Kerman in San Leandro and Mary Lugo in Imperial, California. Finally, what a chore it would have been without the friends who listened to my ideas and shared their own experiences. Thank you to Ruth Baughman, Judy Tesone, Henri Dorsey, Marian Leder, Laura House, Caroline Ariola, and one anonymous friend.

TABLE OF CONTENTS

THE FIRST WARNING SIGNS

WHAT IS HAPPENING TO WESTERN CIVILIZATION? The West is in trouble. It is not just in the United States that cancer, Alzheimer's, and other degenerative diseases are overwhelming people. It is not only in the United States that feelings of depression, guilt, anxiety, and helplessness are widespread. Mental and neurological illnesses have become Europe's biggest health concerns. A major new study found that 38% of the European population suffers from everything from depression to insomnia to dementia.[1] In the United States, roughly one in four middle-aged women are taking antidepressants.[2]

Over 100 years ago, at the beginning of the last century, colonial and missionary doctors knew the diet of the white man was not healthy. Typically, physicians working throughout Africa would report that cancer appeared among natives who had adopted the food of the Europeans, but there was no cancer among those who had retained their traditional diets. For example, Dr. F. P. Fouche had spent six years in South Africa at a hospital serving 14,000 natives. He reported in the British Medical Journal "I never saw a single case of gastric or duodenal ulcer, colitis, appendicitis, or cancer in any form in a native, although these diseases were frequently seen among the white or European population."[3] No one seems to have worried about what would happen to the descendants of these people if each generation continued to eat this unhealthy diet. Now, we are those great, great, great, great grandchildren.

What is it about the Western diet that makes it so dangerous? One clue comes from a 94-year-old woman in a small town. Another clue comes from a scientist studying the longevity of earthworms. The third clue involves the Masai nomads in Africa. We will explore the ways our health and our personalities have changed over time.

We will also look closely at some of the worst, but common, degenerative conditions in Western countries, which includes anorexia, depression, and Alzheimer's disease. What are the specific factors that cause Alzheimer's disease to develop? First, I explain the techniques we used to care for my mother. She knew who I was all the way to the end. We were able to help her avoid many of the worst symptoms of Alzheimer's disease. Then we will learn about others who worked closely with Alzheimer's patients. There is a doctor who searched desperately for a way to help her husband who had early onset Alzheimer's disease. A nurse suspected a vitamin deficiency was causing Alzheimer's-like symptoms. Finally, a group of nuns, members of the Sisters of Notre Dame, volunteered to be tested yearly for Alzheimer's disease, and then they donated their brains for autopsy in what is known as the Nun Study. These people all provide pieces of the Alzheimer's puzzle. When you see how the pieces fit together, you will understand how to protect yourself and how to help someone who has this terrible disease.

Personality is affected just as much as our physical health by generations on the Western diet.[4] College students are experiencing more anxiety and have less empathy than previous generations.[5] An important European study recently found that there has been a doubling of depressive episodes among women since the 1970s.[6] As you read, you will find many examples of how our personalities have changed. If one group becomes obsessed with the moral imperative of their programs while people on the opposing side have become more aggressive and determined, then compromise is a thing of the past. If many women are filled with anxiety and helplessness, while most men do not share their anxiety, men and women will tend to vote for different candidates. Thus, there are political ramifications to the changes in personality discussed in this book as well as implications for the family and for personal fulfillment.

No one doubts that five generations of humans raised on natural food and clean air would be healthier than we are today. Why didn't we sense our danger, break out of our cages, and insist on living a healthy life style early in the last century?

1. Change happened slowly.

2. Improvements in sanitation and control of infectious diseases made it appear that we were getting healthier.

3. It is not the first generation to eat devitalized food that suffers the consequences. It is the children of that generation.

4. There is more money to be made from sick people than from healthy people.

5. A comfortable lifestyle and goodies made from processed milk, grain, and sugar are just too tempting.

By 1930, there were disquieting signs of a decline in health. Would Americans see the danger they were in? Dentists were becoming alarmed over rampant tooth decay and crooked, crowded teeth. History shows that so-called "primitive" people had beautiful, healthy teeth, but that most civilized populations had dreadful teeth.

Researchers conducted studies on the causes of dental decay. Dr. Weston Price, D.D.S. saw these problems in his own dental practice. He thought that it made more sense to study the people that had excellent teeth than it did to study groups that already had wretched teeth. Perhaps he could discover the secrets of these healthy people.

Dr. Price's quest led him around the world to study 14 different isolated groups including the Swiss and Celtic peoples of Europe, Eskimos and Indians of North America, Polynesians and Melanesians in the Pacific islands, tribes in Eastern and Central Africa, the Maori of New Zealand, the Aborigines of Australia, and the Indians of Peru and the Amazon Basin. His research occurred at a pivotal moment in history when it was still possible to find isolated groups and, at the same time, find members of the same ethnic group exposed to the modern way of life for a generation or more. This enabled Dr. Price to observe the health of people living on their traditional diet compared with changes that took place in members of the same group after they had been living on a diet of processed foods.

In the 1930s, there were still small enclaves of people virtually untouched by modern civilization even in Europe. The Loetschental Valley in Switzerland is almost enclosed by three impenetrable mountains, so these people had never been conquered because just a few men could defend the pass into the valley by setting off an artificial landslide. The rugged terrain and the threat of landslides made ordinary commerce impossible. However, in 1930, the 11-mile Loetschberg Tunnel was completed. This enabled Dr. Price to travel to this valley in 1931.

At the altitude of the Loetschental Valley, the winters are long and harsh, but the summers are beautiful. Alpine flowers and lush, green grass filled the valleys. Here Dr. Price found a community of about 2,000 people still living as they and their ancestors had for centuries. They did not have a doctor or a dentist because there was not enough need for them. There was not a jail or a policeman either! All the children were required to attend school for six months and help with the farming for the other six months of the year. Dr. Price was deeply impressed by their lack of materialism, their reverence for God, and their sense of community, as well as their fine physiques.[7]

The diet of these isolated Swiss depended heavily on dairy products. The milk produced during the summer when the cows were eating lush, fast growing grass was very rich and high in vitamin content. This milk would then be used to produce cheese that sustained the people during the winter months. The nutrition of the growing boys and girls consisted largely of a slice of whole rye bread and a piece of summer-made cheese. This was eaten with the fresh milk from goats or cows. Meat was eaten about once a week. Vegetables were eaten primarily in the summer.[8] Note: this milk was not pasteurized or homogenized. It was not skim milk. It was whole, raw milk.

Dr. Price was primarily concerned with the quality of the teeth and dental structures of the groups he studied. He physically examined the teeth, saved a saliva sample, and photographed each subject. He collected voluminous data. He obtained food for chemical analysis and recorded detailed information about daily menus. His wife, Florence, assisted Dr. Price on these trips, and his book is dedicated to her. Much of this information still exists and is being archived by The Price-Pottenger Nutrition Foundation, www.ppnf.org.

Dr. Price studied the teeth of children from several isolated mountain valleys. He found that of the 4,280 teeth he examined, only 3.4% showed signs of tooth decay. This was in sharp contrast to the conditions he found among the Swiss eating a modernized diet. In the large population centers of Switzerland, dental caries were a major problem. At the time of Dr. Price's visit, estimates suggested that 95% to 98% of the people had dental caries.[9] In one large group, 25% of all of the teeth of the children already had tooth decay and only 4% of the children did not have any tooth decay. He also found that the teeth were often irregular and the dental arches had narrowed.[10] The dental arch is the part of the skull that holds the upper teeth. When the arch narrows, the face tends to look thin.

Before the discovery of antibiotics, tuberculosis was associated with an increase in dental caries. Dr. Price found that those whose health had declined to the point that they were susceptible to tooth decay were also susceptible to tuberculosis. Among the groups that he studied, tuberculosis was a widespread and tragic problem. However, he found that those who stayed on their natural, traditional diets almost never succumbed to the disease. Many Americans think of tuberculosis as one of those diseases that decimated the Native-American population. They don't realize that this disease was also tragic for people of European stock. While he was in Switzerland, Dr. Price visited Dr. Rollier, a renowned tuberculosis specialist, in his clinic in Leysin, Switzerland. Dr. Rollier had the general supervision of about 3,500 patients. Dr. Price asked him how many of his patients came from the isolated alpine villages. Not one came from the areas still using a traditional diet. All of the patients came from the Swiss plains and a few from other countries where a modern diet was being eaten.[11]

Dr. Price concluded:

> High immunity to dental caries, freedom from deformity of the dental arches and face, and sturdy physiques with high immunity to disease were

all found associated with physical isolation, and with forced limitation in selection of foods. This resulted in a very liberal use of dairy products and whole-rye bread, in connection with plant foods, and with meat served about once a week.

The individuals in the modernized districts were found to have widespread tooth decay. Many had facial and dental arch deformities and much susceptibility to diseases. These conditions were associated with the use of refined cereal flours, a high intake of sweets, canned goods, sweetened fruits, chocolate, and a greatly reduced use of dairy products.[12]

Where else in Western Europe could an isolated group be found? On some islands! On the Islands of the Outer Hebrides off the coast of Scotland, Weston Price found Celtic people living as they had for generations. These rugged islands extend as far north as the southern part of Greenland and are in the path of North Atlantic storms. The soil is so poor that there are almost no trees and cattle don't mature and reproduce properly. It took great effort and ingenuity to grow some scruffy oats. Deposits of peat, formed from the dead plants of past centuries, were cut and used as fuel. Some small, very hardy sheep were raised. Fishing was the principal occupation and seafood was abundant. There were many lobsters, crabs, oysters, and clams. An important and very popular dish was cod's head stuffed with chopped cod's liver and oatmeal.[13]

The Isle of Lewis had a population of about 20,000. The only large town was the port of Stornoway with a population of about 8,000 including the fishermen who came into port on weekends. In Stornoway, one could buy angel food cake, white bread, and other white-flour products, marmalades, canned vegetables, sweetened fruit juices, and jams. All kinds of goodies were in the store windows. Once away from the town, in the interior and along the coasts, these things were not available. Dr. Price found that in these isolated areas, the teeth of the children had a "very high degree of perfection." Of the teeth that Dr. Price examined, only 1.3% showed any signs of tooth decay.[14] He found that dental caries were "very extensive" in the modernized area. Even worse, in the town, the younger generation did not show as much resistance to tuberculosis as their ancestors. A hospital was being built to care for tubercular patients.[15]

After studying the isolated Celtic people off the coast of Scotland who still followed their traditional lifestyle, Weston Price saw that they had great stamina and superb physiques. He was particularly taken with several women dressed in oilskin suits and rubber boots working at the fish cleaning benches from early morning until late at night. On Sunday, he saw them again. This time they were taking an important role in the leading church. These women lived on a rugged island and had to cope with the treacherous storms and the penetrating, cold fog of the north Atlantic. Dr. Price marveled at their "Gentleness, refinement, and sweetness of character."[16]

According to Dr. Price, it is surprising how much change can take place in one or two generations:

> The change in the two generations was illustrated by a little girl and her grandfather on the Isle of Skye. He was the product of the old regime, and about eighty years of age. He was carrying the harvest from the fields on his back when I stopped him to take his picture. He was typical of the stalwart product raised on the native foods. His granddaughter had pinched nostrils and a narrowed face. Her dental arches were deformed and her teeth crowded. She was a mouth breather. She had the typical expression of the result of modernization after the parents had adopted the modern foods of commerce, and abandoned the oatcake, oatmeal porridge, and seafoods.[17]

Dr. Price summarized his findings:

A dietary program competent to build stalwart men and women and rugged boys and girls is provided the residents of these barren Islands, with their wind and storm-swept coasts, by a diet of oats used as oatcake and oatmeal porridge together with fish products, including some fish organs and eggs. A seriously degenerated stock followed the displacement of this diet with a typical modern diet consisting of white bread, sugar, jams, syrup, chocolate, coffee, some fish without livers, canned vegetables, and eggs.[18]

You can see where this is headed. In one isolated group after another, the people were strong and healthy with great strength and stamina as long as they consumed their traditional diet. Their immunity to disease was high. Even cancer was not a problem. The first generation to be tempted by white flour and sugar did not bear the full consequences. However, the children of this generation were often devastated by disease.[19] So what would happen in the following generation? *Nutrition and Physical Degeneration* by Weston A. Price is one of the most fascinating and profoundly significant books of the twentieth century.

In the prologue to the 50th anniversary edition of his book, some of Dr. Price's research was summarized:

The diets of the healthy primitives Price studied were diverse. Some were based on seafood, some on domesticated animals, some on game, and some on dairy products. Some contained almost no plant foods while others contained a variety of fruits, vegetables, grains, and legumes. In some, mostly cooked foods were eaten, while in others many foods, including animal foods, were eaten raw. However, these diets shared several underlying characteristics. None contained any refined or devitalized foods such as white sugar and flour, canned foods, pasteurized or skimmed milk, and refined and hydrogenated vegetable oils. All diets contained animal products of some sort and all included some salt. Preservation methods among primitive groups included drying, salting, and fermenting. All of which preserve and even increase nutrients in our food.[20]

GENERATION TO GENERATION

WESTON PRICE STUDIED THE FIRST GENERATION to eat processed food and the children of that generation. What would happen if people continued to eat an inadequate diet for generation after generation? There have been animal studies that investigated generational changes. Probably the most well known is the cat study done by Francis M. Pottenger, Jr., M.D. Dr. Pottenger had observed that cats were much healthier if they ate raw meat instead of cooked meat. He decided to study how different the next generation and the generation after that would be if they had only cooked foods. Note: the metabolism of cats and humans is different, so exact correlations cannot be made.

Starting in 1932, Dr. Pottenger conducted a ten-year experiment to determine the effects of heat-processed food on cats. One group of cats was used as a control group. These cats were fed an optimal diet of two-thirds raw meat, one-third raw milk, and cod liver oil. The breeding males were always from this healthy group and were of proven fertility, so the experimental results primarily reflect the health of the mother cats.

The deficient cats were fed a diet of two-thirds cooked meat, one-third raw milk, and cod liver oil.[21] When the meat was heated, all of the enzymes were destroyed. We now know that enzymes are essential for the health of humans, cats, and all other animals. Enzymes are found in raw fruits and vegetables, as well as in meat. However, the particular enzymes and other life-giving factors in raw meat need further study.

The effects of the deficient diet on the ability of the cats to reproduce were really quite sad. The cats had increasing difficulty with their pregnancies, and many of them failed to become pregnant altogether. Miscarriages became very common. The birth of the kittens became difficult, and many female cats died during labor. The average birth weight of the kittens of the cats fed cooked-meat was only 100 grams. Many of the kittens were born dead or were too frail to nurse. When the researchers used a foster mother to attempt saving kittens born to a mother who couldn't nurse them, the kittens were still too frail to survive. The cats on a raw-meat diet had kittens with an average birth weight of 119 grams. The cats in the healthy, raw-meat group had little difficulty reproducing. Miscarriages were rare. The litters averaged five kittens, and the mother cats were able to nurse them without difficulty.[22]

Cats on the cooked-meat diets displayed signs of diseases not seen in the control group. There were heart problems, nearsightedness and farsightedness, and hypothyroidism. Other complications included infections of the kidney, the liver, the bladder, the testes, and the ovaries. Also common was arthritis, inflammation, and many other conditions. As mentioned, antibiotics were still not available at the time of these studies. Many of the cats in the cooked-meat group died from infections. By the third generation, the cats were so unhealthy that none survived beyond six months, and they did not reproduce themselves. The study ended with the third generation.[23] Note: you may wonder why pet cats that eat canned cat food don't seem to have these problems. It is very hard to keep a cat in. They get out and manage to do a little hunting on their own. Some breeders of show cats who keep their cats carefully confined have seen some of the same problems that showed up in the Pottenger study and are very interested in his research.[24]

Over the course of the 10-year study, 900 cats were involved. Six hundred of these had individual, recorded health histories. After the cats died, autopsies were performed. Meticulous care was taken in conducting the autopsies. Dr. Pottenger worked with Alvin G. Foord, M.D., professor of pathology at the University of Southern California and the pathologist at the Huntington Memorial Hospital in Pasadena.[25]

In the results of the studies, many technical details are provided regarding the teeth and the skull. In general, there was a narrowing of the dental arch so that the teeth became crowded and crooked in the cats on a deficient diet. Their faces tended to become longer and narrower. By the third generation, some had a smaller skull or a larger brain case with a smaller face. It is also interesting that their long bones tended to lengthen and become smaller in diameter. Their bones also became more porous.[26]

Knowing that people's jaws became too narrow on a diet of white flour and sweets or that mother cats died in labor on a diet of processed food doesn't disturb us as much as doctors Price and Pottenger expected it would. We have learned to cope with some of these consequences. After all, we can pull out a few teeth and wear braces if the jaw gets too narrow. Babies can be born by caesarian section if a mother's pelvis is not broad enough. Antibiotics can be used to fight infections. Perhaps taking one pill a month will take care of porous bones. Yet we have a dreadful sense that something profoundly dangerous is undermining our society. We do not understand our own children. Each generation is getting weaker. Personalities are changing. Our ability to learn and remember is being taken from us. There is an epidemic of degenerative diseases.

What is the connection between our modern diet and changes in personality and degenerative diseases? Is it the immune system? Is it the digestive system? Probably the most significant observations from Dr.

Pottenger's research have to do with what happened to the immune systems of the cats on a deficient diet. By the third generation, they all had allergies. Allergies are a symptom of a poorly functioning immune system.

Allergies to milk were common among the second and third generation cats. An example is given of a cat that itched so much that it rubbed the fur off its buttocks. When milk was removed from its diet, the symptoms cleared. The cats on a raw-meat diet showed no signs of allergies. However:

> In giving cats cooked meat and milk, they develop all kinds of allergies. They sneeze, wheeze, and scratch. They are irritable, nervous, and do not purr. First deficient generation allergic cats produce second-generation kittens with greater incidence of allergies, and by the third generation, the incidence is almost 100 percent. When second generation allergic animals are bred after being returned to an optimum raw food diet, their allergy symptoms begin to diminish and by the fourth generation, some cats show no evidences of allergy.[27]

The cats did not respond when they were suddenly given a chance to return to their natural diet because too many generations had been on a deficient diet. The number of those with allergies had increased from 5%

in the first generation to more than 95% in the third generation. It required three to four generations of cats raised on a healthy diet of two-thirds raw foods to reverse the damage done by three generation of poor nutrition.[28]

Here is another important observation:

> The intestinal tracts of the allergic cats proved particularly remarkable at autopsy. Measurements of the length of the gastrointestinal tracts of several hundred normal and deficient adult cats were compared. The measurement started at the epiglottis and included the esophagus, the stomach, duodenum, jejunum, and the colon to the rectum. In the average normal cat, the intestinal tract was approximately 48 inches long; in some of the allergic cats, the intestinal tracts measured as long as 72 to 80 inches. These elongated tracts lacked tissue tone and elasticity.[29]

From the Pottenger cat study, you should remember:

1. On a deficient diet, each generation gets weaker.
2. After several generations on a deficient diet, almost all the animals had allergies.
3. There may be a connection between the gastrointestinal tract and allergies.

For the complete details of the Pottenger cat studies, read *Pottenger's Cats: A Study in Nutrition* by Francis M. Pottenger, Jr. Reprints of the original articles by Dr. Pottenger are also available at www.ppnf.org.

STIMULUS AND WITHDRAWAL: HIDDEN ALLERGIES

WHEN DID AMERICANS FIRST BEGIN TO WORRY about allergies? Until the middle of the 19th century, allergies were practically unknown to the general public. According to some medical authorities, hay fever was an "Exceedingly rare occurrence." Asthma and hay fever were the first allergic symptoms that people observed. Soon after the Civil War, the roller flourmill was invented and white flour was produced. This started the sad cascade of consequences that have already been discussed. By the end of the century, hay fever was increasing. The elites went to lovely resorts in the mountains or at the seashore to escape this rather fashionable ailment. Hay fever had become the fourth most common form of chronic disease and a major public health concern in the United States by the 1930s.[30]

Most people who went to an allergist for their hay fever were treated with antigen injections for pollens, molds, and dusts. This became popular in the United States because of the large amounts of ragweed hay fever.

Most clinical allergists limited their practice to giving skin tests and shots for such conditions as hay fever, asthma, and skin rashes based on antigen/antibody reaction theory. Food allergens did not show up reliably with their skin tests, so they tended to downplay the importance of food reactions. They said that anything that could not be treated with their methods was "not allergic."[31]

There is another group of M.D.s with a broader definition of allergies who are concerned about the impact of foods, chemicals, and other environmental factors on their patients. They call themselves clinical ecologists, and they practice environmental medicine. Clinical ecologists focus on identifying and eliminating specific environmental factors.[32] Those of us at the beginning of the 21st century who are trying to recover from over 100 years of processed foods and chemical pollution can learn from the research and experience of these doctors.

There was little interest in food allergies until the late 1920s and 1930s when Albert Rowe, M.D. showed that eliminating wheat, eggs, milk, and other common foods from patient's diets could clear up chronic problems such as migraine headaches, eczema, indigestion, and ulcerative colitis. His patients had not realized that they were reacting to these foods, so they had continued to eat them despite their negative effects. Naturally, this caused chronic health problems. Their allergies had been delayed or hidden.[33] Dr. Herbert Rinkel, M.D. found how to unmask these hidden allergies. His discovery came out of his personal health problems.

Herbert Rinkel had been in World War I as a regimental photographer. After the war, he wanted to be a doctor. Even though he was married, had a son, and no money, he was determined to go to medical school. His father, a farmer in Kansas, sent the family a gross of 144 eggs every week to help them save money on food. During his college years, Rinkel became increasingly ill with a constantly running nose, sore throats, and ear problems. His rhinitis was really severe. When he was using both hands to develop pictures, he would just put his head down and let the ropes of mucous touch the floor. Despite his health problems, he graduated first in his class in medical school.

Rinkel began to suspect that food sensitivity might be behind his rhinitis after he read Rowe's work on elimination diets. He placed six eggs in a blender and drank them. Nothing happened. If anything, he felt better than usual. It wasn't until several years later that he decided to try eliminating eggs from his diet to see if it would help his headache, fatigue, and running nose. He still liked eggs and ate them every day. After two or three days without eggs, he felt better. On the fifth day, he ate a piece of birthday cake that his wife had made for him. He didn't know that there was egg in it. Ten minutes later, he collapsed on the floor. It took several minutes for him to regain consciousness. There were other physicians there for his birthday party who checked his vital signs. They were mystified because there didn't seem to be any reason for him to faint.

When Dr. Rinkel checked with his wife, he found that there had been egg in the birthday cake. He reasoned that staying off a food that he was allergic to for five days had made him hypersensitive to it. He repeated the experiment on himself and had another acute reaction.[34][35] Rinkel discovered that most food reactions are to common foods such as wheat, corn, coffee, eggs, milk, beef, and pork, which are eaten frequently. The patient gets a lift from eating the food he is reacting to. It becomes his or her favorite food. He or she does not realize that the headache or other symptoms that come on a few hours later or even the next day are from eating this food. In order to feel better, he or she eats more of their favorite food. By eliminating this food for four or five days, a patient becomes supersensitive to it. A small amount of the food will cause a strong reaction and unmask a hidden food intolerance or allergy. This is called *masking* or a *masked allergy*.[36] Note: before you try this on yourself or your child, remember that Rinkel ended up on the floor when he tried it. A dangerous reaction is possible. More details will be given later.

By far the most influential doctor in the field of food and chemical allergy is Dr. Theron Randolph, M.D. of

Chicago. Dr. Richard Mackarness, a British doctor and psychiatrist, dedicated his book, *Not All in the Mind,* to Dr. Randolph. Dr. Mackarness stayed with Dr. Randolph and his wife, Tudy, in 1958. He saw the work that Randolph was doing with allergy patients at the Swedish Covenant Hospital, and this revolutionized his own work with depression, schizophrenia, and manic behavior in Great Britain. Dr. Mackarness described Ted Randolph as a tall, thin man resembling that endearing American actor, Jimmy Stewart. Mackarness said that his patients loved him. He had never known a "doctor who took such immense trouble with his patients," and that "he never gives a patient up as hopeless."[37]

Instead of doing carefully controlled and expensive longitudinal studies to determine why more and more people were getting chronic illnesses, Dr. Randolph worked backwards. He took extensive medical histories. He was a very rapid typist. He would sit beside his patient and type their history as they talked. He said that he practiced "poker-faced medicine." He accepted what the patient said without a look or a tone to indicate doubt. A patient who came to him with depression might be surprised when the doctor began asking detailed question about the arthritis that had started 20 years earlier. Had the patient moved to a new house? How was the house heated? Had the patient ever been heavier than he was now? Certain cases were studied in great depth because of the insights into the whole process that Randolph was able to glean. Many of these same patients were also tested in Randolph's Ecology Unit. Here, their hidden food and chemical allergies could be unmasked in a controlled environment. All of this work provided a unique and invaluable database for Randolph to study the way illness had developed over the lifetime of his patients.[38] [39]

Dr. Randolph discovered that people became addicted to the foods and chemicals that they were reacting to. Just as a drug addict gets highs and lows, a food addict gets stimulus and withdrawal reactions. The difference is that the drug addict knows what he is reacting to and why he has highs and lows. Food addicts don't know what they are reacting to or even that they are reacting. As long as he or she is happy, successful, and energetic, a person does not realize that he is on a high, that he is getting a little extra stimulus. It is only when he gets withdrawal symptoms that he realizes that he is sick. That is when he goes to a doctor. Certain patterns began to emerge. Dr. Randolph found that most of his patients had not been sickly all their lives. Indeed, many of them had been attractive, successful people before they became ill. Some had even been dynamic, energetic leaders in their fields earlier in their lives. Some who were thin and depressed had been heavy and outgoing at one point. Some who were obese had been slender until they suddenly started gaining weight.[40]

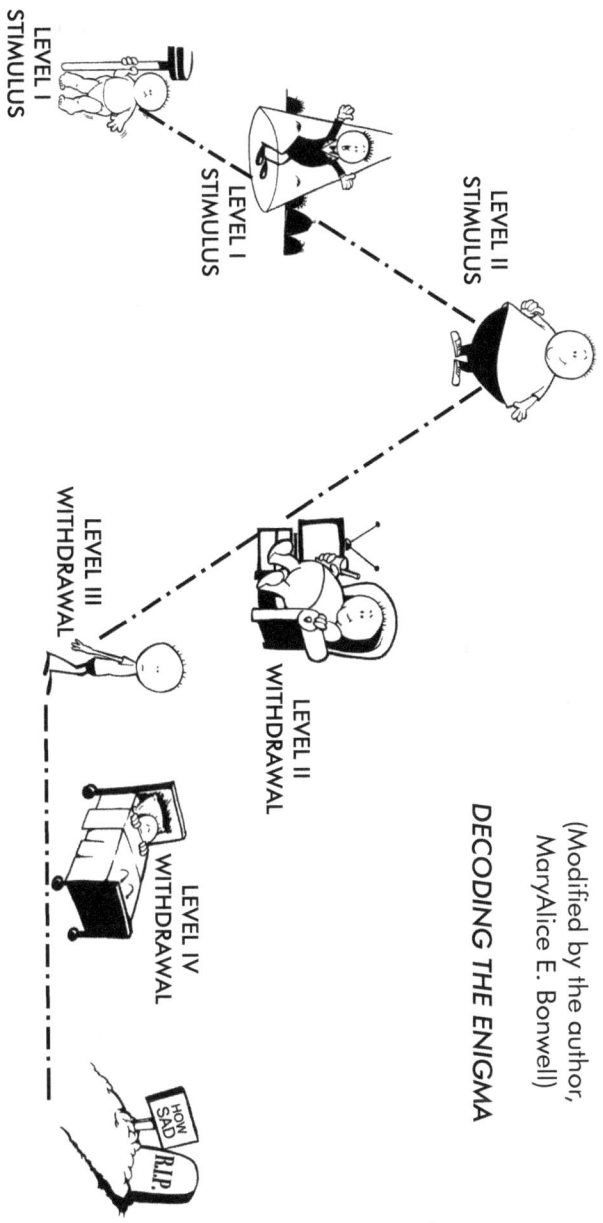

LIFE PATTERNS
A PARTIAL ILLUSTRATION OF THE RANDOLPH PARADIGM

(Modified by the author,
MaryAlice E. Bonwell)

DECODING THE ENIGMA

LEVEL I
STIMULUS

LEVEL I
STIMULUS

LEVEL II
STIMULUS

LEVEL III
WITHDRAWAL

LEVEL II
WITHDRAWAL

LEVEL IV
WITHDRAWAL

HOW
SAD
R.I.P.

© BONWELL   Drawings by Jim Mathenia

Dr. Randolph's most important book for the lay reader is *An Alternative Approach to Allergies,* which was first published in 1980. The subtitle of the book was "The New Field of Clinical Ecology Unravels the Environmental Causes of Mental and Physical Ills." In this book, Randolph lays out levels of stimulus and withdrawal reactions as the symptoms of a hypersensitive immune system become more and more serious. I refer to this framework as the Randolph Paradigm. Most authors who write about Dr. Randolph do not take the time to explain the stages that people go through as they react to specific foods and chemicals in the environment. However, this information is vital in terms of understanding the impact of health on our society and individuals. There are four levels of stimulus reactions and four levels of withdrawal reactions.

At level I stimulus a person is only getting a small amount of stimulus from various foods and other environmental factors, just enough to make him or her attractive. These people are fun to be with. People at this stage are friendly, enthusiastic, and lively. They have a competitive edge over the truly healthy person who is not getting a stimulus. This is where celebrity comes from. These people have charisma. This may appear harmless, but it is the beginning of a long addiction trip, which will end badly.[41]

It is at level II stimulus that the addictive nature of this process really shows itself. A person starts wanting more and more. It may be more food, more alcohol, or more of other stimulants to stay on a high. Both obesity and alcoholism are a problem at this level. A person craves his favorite foods. He even wakes up in the middle of the night and can't go back to sleep until he has a snack of some favorite food. At this stage, a person has the energy and drive to be a successful entrepreneur, a charismatic teacher, or a greatly admired political leader. However, he may become hyperactive, aggressive, and obviously self-centered. This is the effusive and overly aggressive car salesman or the backslapping politician. At this stage, "restless legs" syndrome frequently occurs. In children, this is the stage when hyperactivity and learning disorders become a problem. Most people do not go higher than level II on the stimulus side.[42]

If a level II person does continue up the stimulus side to level III stimulus, he will become so self-centered that he will tend to be indifferent to the thoughts and feelings of others. He appears quite strange and people tend to stay away from him. However, some of these people can keep up a pretense of normality with outsiders. They may appear to be highly dynamic, intense leaders. They make disastrous leaders because of their egomania and poor judgment. They are often anxious and afraid of real or imagined dangers.[43]

At level IV stimulus a person is obviously sick. Dr. Randolph says that this level appears to be just like the manic phase of manic-depression. A person may flail his arms and legs and have convulsions. He may be obsessed by strange, irrational ideas and not know where he is. He may be excited, agitated, enraged, or panicky. His mind may go around in circles, or he may have one-track thoughts.[44]

A person usually doesn't go higher than level II stimulus before he starts down the withdrawal side. Very often, some annoying withdrawal symptoms will be present even when a person is still primarily on the stimulus side. For example, an active and charming level I stimulus person may have some problems with hay fever or constipation. He will ignore these symptoms or just use some over the counter remedies because the lift on the stimulus side makes him feel well overall.

Level I withdrawal reactions include localized physical problems such as a stuffy nose, coughing, asthma, itching, eczema, gas, diarrhea, constipation, and colitis. These are the kinds of reactions that most people think of as "allergies." Dr. Randolph also lists urgency and frequency of urination, and various eye and ear syndromes, including Meniere's syndrome and an impaired sense of smell and taste as problems that occur at level I withdrawal.[45]

At level II withdrawal, there are many physical reactions. Usually they are "systemic" symptoms affecting many parts of the body. Typically, a person is tired. The high energy, which had been a vital part of his or her personality, disappears and is replaced by allergic fatigue. Allergic fatigue is very different from normal fatigue that comes as a result of work and exercise. Allergic fatigue doesn't seem to have a reason and sleep and rest don't seem to help. A person at this level often suffers from painful syndromes such as headaches, neck and backaches, muscle aches, and arthritis. Edema may occur. Cardiovascular symptoms appear at this stage. Randolph mentions a rapid or irregular pulse, tachycardia, arrhythmia, hypertension, phlebitis, anemia, and a tendency toward bruising.[46]

Mental symptoms replace physical symptoms at level III withdrawal. People are often anxious and depressed. This is the stage of mental exhaustion. A person sometimes has difficulty making decisions. He or she may be confused and moody. They might be withdrawn and apathetic with a lack of initiative and ambition. There may be an occasional loss of libido. A person may have trouble in school because of poor memory, attention, and comprehension. These people look normal, but they don't function very well. They are often told that they are hypochondriacs or that their problems are psychosomatic. Dr. Randolph found that when patients were taken off of the foods and chemicals they were reacting to, such "mental" symptoms would clear.[47]

Level IV withdrawal, severe depression, is the end of the line for this whole problem. This stage usually comes on after a super-stimulated phase, as in manic-depressive disease or after the less severe symptoms of level III withdrawal. A patient may be deeply depressed and disoriented. He or she may have paranoid thinking, incontinence, delusions, and hallucinations. Sometimes amnesia and coma may occur.[48]

A person with a hypersensitive immune system changes as he or she goes through life. Typically, young people are on the stimulus side followed by withdrawal reactions at the end of life. The same foods and chemicals that used to give them a lift on the stimulus side makes them feel tired, depressed, and forgetful, or it gives them a headache or arthritis when the withdrawal side becomes dominant. This is why we have the stereotype of the pretty, young teacher, the stout, aggressive, middle-aged teacher, and the burnt out older teacher just hanging on until retirement. These are not three different people, but the same person at different stages of the allergy trip. Another example is the talented and meltingly beautiful young actress, who later in life has to fight obesity or perhaps drugs and alcohol.

What are Randolph's stages of stimulus and withdrawal based on? How much experience did he have? Dr. Randolph lived from 1906 to 1995. He was a practicing allergist in the Midwest, primarily in the Chicago area, for over 50 years beginning in the late 1930s. His bibliography contains close to 400 published scientific articles, which does not even include his many speeches and popular presentations. A complete list of these articles is available in his book, *Environmental Medicine: Beginnings & Bibliographies of Clinical Ecology.* He hospitalized, fasted, and tested over 10,000 individuals in environmentally controlled settings.[49] He carefully recorded and indexed thousands of case histories. Dr. Randolph's papers are now at the Countway Library of Medicine, which is associated with Boston Medical Library and Harvard Medical School.

PATTERNS OF PERSONALITY

MANY OF THE PEOPLE WHO READ DR. RANDOLPH'S work have serious health problems and have not gotten much help from the medical establishment. I was one of those people. In my late thirties, my health collapsed with constant vomiting, confusion, dizziness, and exhaustion. I was a reading specialist too allergic to the chemicals in books to read and too sick to continue teaching. I finally went to live with my mother in a small town in southern California. It was a long road back. Since I was reacting to print, I thought of selling reading boxes to others who were chemically sensitive. I started Safe Haven and sold the Safe Haven Vacuum Reading Box. A small fan in the box sucked the chemicals away from the patient. It really worked quite well. The reason this is important now is that I talked on my 800 line with hundreds of people from all over the country who had serious food and chemical allergies. Because of the Reading Box, I also heard the professional presentations and talked with many people at the annual meetings of the American Academy of Environmental Medicine.

I learned more about the final stages of Environmental Illness by taking care of my aunt and my mother at the ends of their lives. Mother's older sister had Parkinson's disease. We brought her to our home and cared for her during the last two years of her life. After my aunt's death, Mother began to slip into Alzheimer's disease. By using Dr. Randolph's methods, we were able to prevent many of the symptoms of this terrible illness. I write about ways of avoiding Alzheimer's disease later in this book.

Gradually, my health began to improve, although I still had to be very careful of my diet. After about ten years, I was able to return to teaching. I was fortunate in finding a special education position teaching in an elementary school in the town of Imperial, California, just north of El Centro. I also continued to take classes and earned a master's degree in the field of learning handicapped. Of course, as soon as I started teaching again, I realized that many of my students had symptoms such as hyperactivity, poor memory, impulsiveness, and directional confusion that are common among those who are reacting to foods and chemicals.

One afternoon, as I was walking back to my classroom after lunch, I saw a big, heavy, sixth-grade girl mouthing off at a noon supervisor. It came to me that she was obviously level II stimulus. I wondered why we weren't helping her with her reactions to foods and chemicals instead of punishing her. As I unlocked my classroom door, I saw a class of third graders lined up outside their room waiting for their teacher. They were pushing, shoving, and yelling at each other. It came to me that those kids were at level I stimulus. That is why they were so bold and disrespectful in class. The homeless probably fit into this picture on the withdrawal side, I mused. I wondered if there might be a problem in our society for every one of Dr. Randolph's levels of stimulus and withdrawal reactions. Could this be the real reason for the decay in our society?

For the last 25 years, I have been observing how the pieces fit together: how the patterns of personality and the problems of society relate to the changes in health that have taken place over the last century. I thought a lot of people would be writing about this. I have been waiting for a real doctor, or at least a real writer, who could write cleverly and entertainingly, to come forward and explain how the problems of society are related, but it hasn't happened. The enormous crush of daily information seems to have broken all our problems into little bits and magnified the pieces instead of showing us the fundamental causes.

I am writing as a patient, a caregiver, and a teacher. I am not a doctor, nor do I have any background in the sciences. If you are interested in changing any part of your health program based on what I write, be sure to consult with your doctor. I may be totally unaware of some aspects of the problem.

My goal is to show how changes in our health have caused unexpected changes in our personalities and our ability to function. These changes are behind many problems in our society. I will paint, with a broad brush, an overview of connections and relationships. I hope that examples from my experience will trigger examples from your own life.

Most people are reacting to at least some foods and chemicals after a century of processed foods and a polluted environment. Dr. Randolph demonstrated that people get both stimulus and withdrawal reactions when this happens. Both their physical health and their personality are affected. Broken marriages, weight gain, depression, learning disabilities, road rage, bratty kids, drug addiction, and Alzheimer's disease are all part of the picture.

It all starts out innocently enough with a child or young person who seems very outstanding. You might think of this as the Type A personality. He is on the go, loves to multitask, and is great at the computer. He has lots of energy for sports and can keep up with all the other Type A students at school. Let's say that he is reacting to wheat and sugar. He loves his bowl of dry cereal with sugar and milk every morning. He doesn't get bored with the same cereal each day. It is satisfying and tastes great because he is addicted to both wheat and sugar. His parents wish he weren't quite so hyper, but they figure that is just the way kids are. This is level I stimulus. Some people are very lucky. They stay at this stage until late middle age and never realize why they have so much energy. Unfortunately, being at level I stimulus can lead to what I call "Type A gone bad" and "Type A payback" later in life.

Then the weight comes on. It seems like a person used to eat anything they wanted and still stay slender and trim. All of a sudden, they crave food and even looking at a donut will put the pounds on. This is the world of level II stimulus. They still have plenty of energy and drive, but they hate being fat and their aggressiveness may turn people away. This is the stage where alcoholism and learning disabilities become problems. Some children start life at level II stimulus. There are plenty of plump, assertive, little first graders. Some people stay at level II most of their lives and are still fighting the weight problem in their eighties.

Some people continue even further up the stimulus ladder to level III stimulus. This extra stimulus often causes them to be brilliant and talented. However, they begin to lose their connectedness to other human beings. They are often socially awkward. Some will become creative artists or brilliant scientists. Some will join the Geek Squad and help the rest of us with our computers.

A few, at the extremes, may become sociopaths and mass murderers. At level IV stimulus there can be outright mental illness; schizophrenia and autism may occur at this level.

The withdrawal reactions at levels I and II are primarily physical. Level I withdrawal reactions are localized physical problems. At level II, there are systemic symptoms that affect many parts of the body. Thus you can have a happy, energetic, Type A person who has problems with asthma, eczema, or constipation. The heavy, happy, energetic, Type A person at level II is more likely to have heart problems, edema, or arthritis. At level II withdrawal, a person loses the energy that has been such an important part of his personality. Suppose that he loves milk. When he used to drink milk, eat ice cream, or put cream in his coffee, it tasted wonderful and he got a lift. That lift, or extra energy, would last all afternoon until he had more milk with his dinner. After he hits the withdrawal side, milk is his enemy. He still loves milk and it feels good going down, but a few hours later, he feels exhausted. He can barely hang in there to get anything done.

During level III withdrawal, some unexpected changes take place in personality. Symptoms become mental rather than physical. People lose the extra weight they had at level II and become thin. Some of their physical symptoms may disappear, and they become energetic and flexible. Older people at this level often appear to be doing very well. In reality, the problem has just gone to a new level. These people have trouble making decisions. The key symptom is anxiety. As people sink deeper into level III withdrawal, depression becomes the primary problem. In bipolar disorder, a person moves from depression on the withdrawal side to manic behavior on the stimulus side and back again. Depression is becoming more and more common.

Suppose that a little girl is reacting to oranges. She always has orange juice for breakfast, and she likes to have an orange when she gets home from school. She is one of the outstanding children in elementary school. In junior high school, she gains some weight and is very concerned about her appearance. In high school, at level III withdrawal, she manages to lose the weight and becomes very slender and attractive. She tries to eat well and always makes sure that she has an orange or some orange juice every day. She becomes very anxious about her grades even though her parents tell her not to pressure herself. She graduates from high school and sinks into deep depression. She even has suicidal thoughts. She no longer eats so many oranges, but she likes to drink hot water with a little lemon in it. She is always sipping lemon water from a thick mug, which she holds to keep her hands warm. None of her friends or family can conceive of why she is depressed.

In an actual case, no doubt other foods and chemicals would also be involved.

Level IV withdrawal is the end of the line. Alzheimer's disease, Parkinson's disease, and other diseases may belong to this stage.

As we will see later in this book, other factors such as vitamin deficiencies, vascular problems, and difficulty utilizing glucose combine with late stage allergies and food intolerance to cause serious diseases.

A truly healthy person stays about the same all their life, without the highs and lows or the big weight changes that affect the person reacting to foods and chemicals. Both the health and personality of a person with reactions to environmental factors change throughout their lives. Their sense of humor, their self-control, their self-confidence, and even their religious beliefs may change depending on what stage they are experiencing. In the next few chapters, we will examine some of these patterns of personality.

DIRECTIONALITY

THE EFFECTS OF ALLERGIES AND FOOD AND chemical intolerance on personal characteristics first occurred to me while I was taking care of my mother who had Alzheimer's disease. She gradually lost her sense of direction and could not look where I pointed or help herself move into a better position in bed. She didn't know which direction to move her body. At the same time, I was working with children in special education who couldn't tell the difference between the letters *b* and *d*. It struck me that, in both cases, directionality was affected, but in very different ways.

A good sense of direction is a sign of health. Healthy people and those at levels I and II stimulus tend to have an excellent sense of direction. They quickly grasp the lay of the land in a strange city, and they are not afraid to drive to an unfamiliar location. At an unmarked intersection, they know which way to turn. What comes so easily to these people can be difficult or impossible for someone else.

Dr. Randolph identified learning disorders in children, such as attention deficit disorder, as occurring at level II stimulus. I worked with these kinds of children too. The problem that poor readers often have with directionality is interesting because it is so specific. It is directionality in the language area. It is rare to find a child who actually sees everything backward as in mirrored reading, but it is common for children to confuse certain letters such as *b* and *d* or *u* and *n*. (This is considered developmentally normal through first and even second grade). A student might read *ded* for *bed* or *duck* for *back*. A third grader spelled the word *old* as *blo*. He wrote the word backwards and then reversed the *d*. On a test question, one boy read "a *door* has two _____." instead of, "A *bird* has two _____." He read *d* for *b* and guessed at the rest. This same boy would not have trouble finding his mother's car in the parking lot or skateboarding all over town.

In a special education class, usually some students can read words, but they still have great difficulty with comprehension. This may be the "Space Cadet," the one who can't pay attention, forgets, and gets confused. These children are usually at level III withdrawal. They can read *b* and *d*, but often have a very poor general sense of direction. We had a popular game that we usually played at the end of the school year. Each team gained points by directing their team member to locate a city on the classroom wall map using only the terms north, south, east, and west. One fifth grader just couldn't follow his team's hints to go "north, north, north, not south." Finally, they told him to "go up, up, up," but he was still confused. After this happened, I kept him with me to help keep score instead of putting him in an embarrassing position again.

One afternoon, a very pretty, sweet fourth-grade girl, who appeared to be at level III withdrawal, volunteered to take a note over to room 41. When I looked out the window, I saw that she had started in the wrong direction. I went out and pointed her in the right direction. Ten minutes later, I came out of another room and saw her wandering around at the other side of the playground by room 24. I walked with her to deliver the original note to the correct classroom. This room turned out to be only two classrooms away from her homeroom. Later that same afternoon when I was reading with a little second grader, we happened to read a short story called *The Reindeer People* from a Reader's Digest Skill Builder:

> Another special thing about the Lapps is that they never get lost in their travels. They can find a place again, even if they haven't been back to it in years! It's as if they carry a map in their minds.

Children are not the only ones who have these problems. At level III withdrawal, many women have a problem with directionality. They hate to drive to an unfamiliar location. Their families may tease them about losing the car in the parking lot or turning the wrong way after leaving a restaurant.

In the early stage of Alzheimer's disease, a person is in increasing danger of getting lost while driving or getting confused in a crowded shopping mall. When Alzheimer's has progressed to the moderate stage, spatial confusion causes the patient to misjudge distance and direction to the point that driving is no longer safe. In advanced stages, the patient does not know the position of his own body. If a caregiver asks the patient to move forward to help him into a wheelchair, he does not know how to move his body. One of the tests used to diagnose Alzheimer's involves numbers placed randomly on a page. The person being tested is asked to draw a line from one number to the next from the lowest to the highest number. Observers have wondered why this is a difficult task for people with Alzheimer's disease. I suspect that it is because they do not know which direction to move their hand.

Some people with autism have an odd habit of slapping themselves. Temple Grandin, author of *Thinking in Pictures,* explains that some autistic people do not know where their body stops and the world begins. They have serious body boundary problems. They slap themselves to find where their body is. Sometimes they don't know where their legs are if they can't see the legs. She mentions one woman who would bite herself when she was over stimulated by too much noise. The women didn't realize that she was biting her own body. Autism, which may be caused at least in part by food and chemical intolerance, probably has the most extreme forms of spatial dysfunction.[50]

Some autistic people have tried to tell us what they are experiencing when they act in ways that seem inexplicable to us. Temple Grandin, Ph.D. has let us into her world in *Thinking in Pictures and Other Reports from My Life with Autism.* She used her extraordinary visual skills and her empathy for animals to build a career as an animal scientist. She has designed nearly half the livestock-handling facilities in the United States. She also lectures frequently on autism. Her writing is so clear and insightful that it is a must-have book for teachers as well as parents and grandparents of an autistic child. Temple Grandin's book proved to be an invaluable resource for me.

Note: a person who has problems with balance and directionality may be suffering from a vitamin B12 deficiency, which can easily be corrected by supplements or shots if it is caught early enough. Do not ignore these warning signs. Symptoms of vitamin B12 deficiency will be discussed later in this book.

After I started thinking about the ways that our sense of direction changes at different levels of the Randolph paradigm, I began to see that other parts of our personality are also affected by our reactions to foods and chemicals. Our self-control, our ability to pay attention, our closeness to each other, our desire to communicate, and even our sense of humor can be influenced by our reactions. Let's begin by discussing our sense of humor.

HUMOR

WE EXPECT OUR FRIENDS TO HAVE A GOOD SENSE of humor. It is an attractive part of our personalities that we share with each other. A healthy person uses humor to keep from taking himself too seriously. However, as more and more people have been overstimulated, humor has become louder and cruder, and there has been a coarsening of our society. With more stimuli, humor takes on a mean, spiteful quality and some who are over stimulated to the point of being sociopaths think it is hugely funny when they hurt someone. At some stages, a sense of humor is greatly diminished or even disappears.

With children and young teens at level I stimulus there is a lot of silliness over nothing. Little things are very funny. When a few teenagers get together, they feel comfortable laughing and being silly over very little. However, many older teenagers and young adults have a sense of humor that is bolder and cruder than earlier generations.

Most people at level II stimulus are a lot of fun to be with. They have a good sense of humor, and they love to laugh. However, at this level, humor tends to becomes more broad, louder, and coarser. A person likes to "push the envelope" and takes a wicked pride in saying something not quite acceptable. He may just change one or two letters in what everyone knows is a four-letter word. "Potty humor" may seem very funny. It is interesting that in Tourette syndrome, which probably occurs at level III stimulus, obscenities and foul language burst out of a person's mouth without his being able to control it. Screaming and foul language are often a part of the violent tantrums thrown by bipolar children.[51]

Some people at level II stimulus think they are very entertaining. They may laugh loudly at their own jokes, even when those around them don't respond. Slapstick is a scream. Advertisers have picked up on this trait. For example, humor is widely used in Super Bowl ads to appeal to sports fans. One ad for a stock-trading firm has the office workers jump around like gorillas every time the boss's back is turned. One airline advertises that you can get a shorter, direct flight so that you won't have to sit too long next to one of these jokers.

More and more, aggressive people with obnoxious attitudes happily go beyond what is socially appropriate. They see edgy, raunchy comedy as just being what people are really thinking. Other aggressive people on the stimulus side say "right on!"

As a person becomes even more stimulated and moves into level III stimulus, humor becomes twisted.

He thinks it is funny when somebody gets hurt. At a moderate level, he may take pleasure in annoying other people. I was standing in line at the service desk. The man ahead of me asked me why I was there.

I told him, "To pick up my computer."

He asked, "You mean you're going to lift it up and carry it?"

"A friend came with me," I replied.

He continued, "You mean your friend is going to pick up the computer?"

I answered, "We will each pick up a corner."

And on and on!

He was mildly amused at annoying me, and he also enjoyed showing off his superior mind.

One of the techie humor books found at *thinkgeek. com* was *Prank University.* This was described as being "one hundred essential pranks for really getting even."

Teenage boys who are addicted to video games sometimes think it is very funny when the characters get hurt. The TV program, *Intervention,* shows actual film of people with drug, alcohol, and other addictions and tries to get them to go for treatment. One young man didn't care about anything in life except playing video games. His mother said that he showed more emotion when he was playing the games than he ever did in real life. He thought it was very funny when game characters got hurt. He stuck his fist in his mouth to show how the bullet had gone in a character's mouth and killed him. "It was really cool," he said and laughed loudly.

At the extremes of the stimulus continuum, where we see psychotic behavior, a person actually thinks it is funny when somebody else gets hurt. The D.C. Snipers, John Allen Muhammad and Lee Boyd Malvo, killed ten and wounded three in a random shooting spree that terrorized residents of the Washington D. C. area. Malvo fired shots from the trunk of a battered, old Chevy while Muhammad drove the car and planned the attacks. Malvo laughingly described some of the shootings to police detectives. He gloated about the killings in taped conversations. He chuckled as he remembered how one man, after being struck by the bullet, had fallen while the lawnmower he had been pushing continued to move along.[52]

Columbine High School mass murderers Dylan Klebold and Eric Harris killed 13 people and wounded over 20 others in a vicious shooting rampage before killing themselves. They had honed their shooting skills at a firing range in Denver. According to "Final Report" shown on National Geographic TV, they had taken video of themselves shooting at trees and bowling pins. They gleefully held a badly smashed bowling pin up to the camera and laughingly imagined what that bullet would have done inside someone's brain. One of the students who saw them taunting and killing other students in the library said, "They were kind of whopping it up and just having a good time." A to-do-list in their own handwriting was found. At the end they had written "have fun."

Food and chemical reactions can also reduce a person's sense of humor, and in Alzheimer's and autism, humor disappears entirely. Going down the withdrawal side, a person at level III withdrawal has a diminished sense of humor. A woman at this level may seem rather prim. She enjoys quiet humor and loves the cute things that animals do, but she is offended by loud aggressive humor and may not get the point of jokes that make other people laugh. In his battle against feminism, Rush Limbaugh likes to use the term "feminazi." Most people find this to be a clever and humorous pairing of terms even if they don't agree with him. However, a woman on the withdrawal side may find it humorless and mean spirited.

On Valentine's Day, the rather aggressive woman host on Sirius Radio Classical Favorites suggested that listeners tune to the humor channel for special valentine humor. She wondered if you had ever wished that you could turn cupids arrows back on him and get him in his little diapered butt. To her, this was highly amusing, but to a level III withdrawal person enjoying classical music, it would strike an unwelcome rough note that was more crude than funny.

People who are either being stimulated or depressed by the foods and chemicals they are exposed to have no idea that these reactions are changing their personality. What could be more a matter of free will or choice than what we laugh at? Yet, there is a physical factor, actually a health factor, which is fundamental to our appreciation of humor.

COMMUNICATION
AND RELATIONSHIPS

LET'S LOOK AT SOME OTHER ASPECTS OF personality. People at level I stimulus tend to be warm and friendly. It is easy for them to relate to others. They love to talk with friends. This is the teenager talking for hours on the phone, chatting with friends while shopping, or whispering in the classroom. This may also be little Miss Celebrity who enjoys being the center of attention. She would love to be a cheerleader or in the talent show. She likes to be looked at and have an audience. If bare midriffs or short skirts are in style, she will be comfortable showing them off.

The desire to have an audience has become more common as each generation has become weaker, and in some, any sense of modesty or privacy has disappeared. People have no shame about undressing and putting their pictures on the Internet. On social networking sites, underage girls post provocative photos of themselves in next to nothing. On the message boards, they brag about their sexual experimentations.

At level II stimulus, people are full of emotion. Their joy, hugs, tears, and anger are all on the surface, ready to spill over. Their all-enveloping hugs often do not express commitment, or even lasting concern, but merely the happiness of the moment. Despite their weight, producers of game shows and reality TV frequently select these people as contestants because they bring emotion to the camera. Some of these people love to be the center of attention, and they will often clown around or play the jokester at parties. Some have an "in your face" attitude about how they look, such as the fat woman who wears shorts to the company picnic.

People at level II stimulus usually love to talk. Some are very articulate and become excellent public speakers and outstanding orators.

However, others just never stop talking. This is the "babbling brook." You can't get them to stop. First, the teacher moves one student away and then another, until he is all by himself, but still Joe is talking. The husband goes outside to weed the garden. At least out there he can get away from the incessant chatter! The other teachers avoid her so that they won't get trapped into an endless conversation.

People on the withdrawal side like to talk, but they usually don't want to get up in front of other people. They feel very comfortable talking with friends who share their lifestyle and political views. Those with environmental illness can go on endlessly about their symptoms and the healing techniques they are trying.

One of my close EI friends, a very sweet person who has probably been a level III withdrawal person most of her life, told me years ago that she hadn't gone to college because she would have had to take speech. That had stuck with me because it seemed like such a loss. I recently asked her to tell me more about what had happened. It seems that as a high school senior she had been required to give current events reports in her social studies class. She was very afraid of getting up in front of the class. She looked for the shortest article in the paper and hoped desperately that no one would ask a question. Each time she fell apart inside and could hardly talk. In her yearbook, one adjective was placed under the picture of each senior. Her word was "timid." She applied to San Diego State and was accepted. She passed the entrance exam. A postcard came with her class schedule, and it included speech. She knew she couldn't do it, and she asked her parents to help her go to secretarial school.

Some unexpected things begin to happen to our ability to communicate and to relate to others as we climb the stimulus ladder. You may notice that I am speaking primarily about men. This is because more men tend to be on the stimulus side and more women go down the withdrawal side. More men are entrepreneurs. More men love to watch football. More men are geeks. More men are serial killers. More boys have autism. Going down the withdrawal side, more women suffer from Environmental

Illness, autoimmune diseases, and depression. Finally, more women have Alzheimer's disease.

A person who is reacting to foods and chemicals, and perhaps electro-magnetic fields, can be overstimulated enough to reach level III stimulus. Here the symptoms are primarily mental rather than physical. Thinking abilities are stimulated. A person may be brilliant and talented, but this comes at the expense of the emotional part of life. In marriage, where loving, caring, and communicating are central to the relationship, this may play a bigger role than we have previously realized.

In a perceptive article, "Why Women Leave Men," Willard F. Harley, Jr., Ph.D. writes about the real reasons that women ask for a divorce. Surprisingly few women leave because of serious factors such as physical abuse, infidelity, and alcoholism. Almost all of the reasons that women divorce their husbands can be grouped under the heading of neglect. This includes indifference and failing to communicate. Women have confided:

> "We're like ships passing in the night, he goes his way, and I go mine."

> "My husband is no longer my friend."

> "My husband has become a stranger to me; I don't even know who he is anymore."

"He lives his life as if we weren't married; he rarely considers me."

"He doesn't show any interest in me or what I do."

To a man who is working hard to support his family, this may seem like trivial carping, but loving, caring, and sex are the glue that hold marriage together. In some cases, a man has merely been careless and inconsiderate or has allowed his career to consume all of his time and energy. However, if a man's ability to feel love and connectedness has gradually seeped away, he is usually unaware of any change and doesn't empathize with his wife's need for closeness. The women who talk with Dr. Harley usually despair about getting their husbands to understand what is wrong.[53] Could it be that, at some level, these women sense that the emotion they are searching for simply isn't there?

At level II stimulus, we saw a heavy person with excess emotion on display for everyone to see. At level III stimulus, we usually see a thin person who is more withdrawn and has diminished emotions. Instead of being eager to talk and enjoying center stage, the level III stimulus person loses his desire to communicate and would rather not talk. He doesn't like to be looked at. He may not want his picture taken. His wife may complain that her husband just sits in front of the TV or reads a book and doesn't talk with her. If he gets deeper into level III, he may turn the lack of a desire to talk into a weapon and give his wife, or some other family member, the silent treatment. His sense of hearing, sight, and even touch may become hypersensitive. He may wear dark glasses when others don't need them. He may refuse to eat with the family because he can't stand the sound of a person chewing food.

As a person goes even higher on the level III stimulus scale, he tends to miss social cues and become a self-described geek. Such a person is very smart, but he doesn't relate well to other people. From the *New Hacker's Dictionary* by Eric S. Raymond, we can gain some insight into how people are affected as they become more and more stimulated by environmental factors. Raymond paints a portrait of J. Random Hacker, which is based on the comments of about a hundred Usenet respondents. (Note: according to Raymond, a hacker is someone who enjoys, and is even obsessed by, exploring the details of computer programs and how to stretch their capabilities. Those who maliciously break into computer programs to commit theft and vandalism are called crackers. Hackers despise these vandals.)[54]

J. Random Hacker is intelligent, intense, and either too thin or too heavy. Most are too thin and 90% are male. He tends to be self-absorbed and have little ability to identify emotionally with other people. A hacker is often very well read and has a fund of knowledge that he could share, but he usually doesn't have any urge to communicate. After a few words, he is likely to turn back to his computer.[55]

Hackers tend to dress in the same scruffy, casual way and have many of the same interests, but Raymond makes the point that hackers don't get that way by imitating each other. There seems to be something within their personality that makes them that way. One trait he mentions tends to corroborate my contention that this type of personality stems from being on the stimulus side of food and chemical intolerance. According to Raymond, "Almost all hackers have terribly bad handwriting."[56] Doris Rapp, M.D., well-known clinical ecologist and pediatrician, has found that food and chemical reactions can affect handwriting. As she is testing a child, she will often have him write his name or color a picture from a coloring book. A child who can color within the lines and print his name neatly before the testing starts often loses these skills when he reacts to an antigen. His coloring may become scribbles. His letters are poorly formed and his name may be illegible. Fascinating examples of changes in handwriting during allergy testing can be found in the book *Is This Your Child's World?* by Dr. Rapp.[57]

At stimulus level IV, emotions have become truncated. The softer emotions of love, concern, and remorse have disappeared, but fear, anger, and lust remain. This is where we find the psychopaths. Despite the horrific things they have done, they feel no remorse. Even in the courtroom, where it is a matter of their own life or death, they do not show remorse. Biography Channel profiled Richard Ramirez, the Night Stalker, who is one of the most heinous serial rapists and murderers in the twentieth century. He said, "Most killers in general have a dead conscience." As he leafed through crime photos in court, he clearly relished the details all over again. When parts of bodies were shown, he would laugh and giggle. The dislike of being looked at becomes extreme at this level. Ramirez told one terrified woman, "Don't look at me. If you look at me again, I'll shoot you." Another victim was found with her eyes gouged out and the bloody sockets empty.[58] [59]

At level IV stimulus, some of the most common symptoms found in autistic children involve their lack of any desire to communicate. They prefer to be alone. They have abnormal speech or no speech, and they do not make eye contact. They do not relate emotionally to their parents or their siblings. One autistic, four-year-old boy, when asked at the family breakfast table if he wanted waffles or pancakes, replied, "Purple." Then he hit everyone within reach and retreated into one of his obsessions: taking everything out of the refrigerator and then putting everything back in, emptying, filling, emptying, and filling. When they spoke to him and called his name in various situations, he was so unresponsive that they had him tested for deafness.[60]

Temple Grandin, whom I referred to earlier, writes that fear and anxiety are the predominant emotions of many autistic people. At a conference, one man told her that he only feels three emotions: fear, sadness, and anger. He has no joy. She explains that she does have emotions, but they are more shallow and child-like than a normal adult. She becomes very angry if people abuse cattle, but if they stop abusing the animals, the anger quickly passes. She can see that a flower is pretty or a mountain is big, but she doesn't feel an emotional response. She says that she does not know "what complex emotion in a human relationship is. I only understand simple emotion such as fear, anger, happiness, and sadness."[61]

Warm and friendly to distant and uncommunicative, our personalities are affected by our reactions to foods and chemicals. Good health is fundamental to a healthy personality and our ability to relate to others.

ATTENTION

FOR CENTURIES, WE HAVE BEEN PAYING attention to each other. We listened to the person we were talking with. We focused on the meaning of the book we were reading. We didn't think this was anything special. Paying attention was just another human ability that we took for granted. Now we are finding that a hypersensitive immune system can change our ability to pay attention. People with food and chemical intolerance are affected differently at the different levels.

Today's overstimulated young people don't pay attention to one thing at a time. No, they multitask. They are geniuses with computers, cell phones, and other electronic gadgets. They love to talk on the cell phone, check their email, and keep track of their bids on eBay all at the same time. They feel busy, connected, alive, and very smart. They usually think that multitasking started with them and the tech revolution. Actually, this behavior type was spotted a couple of generations earlier in the 1960s.

In the 1960s, two well-known cardiologists, Meyer Friedman, M.D. and Ray Rosenman, M.D. noticed that many of their heart patients always seemed to be in a hurry. These patients felt pressured by time. They walked rapidly and tried to do more than one thing at once. Such a patient might shave and dictate letters into his portable tape recorder while driving to work. Someone who spoke slowly might irritate him. He might be annoyed, even angry, if the person ahead of him drove too slowly. These people tended to be assertive or aggressive, and in advanced cases, there was a kind of free-floating hostility. The two doctors called this "hurry sickness." They found that "hurry sickness" was a better predictor of heart attacks than blood pressure, weight, or other factors that are usually monitored.[62]

The name "hurry sickness" was rolled over into "Type A Behavior," and Drs. Friedman and Rosenman published *Type A Behavior and Your Heart* in 1974. This book became a huge bestseller. Some people tried to change their attitude, but that didn't seem to prevent heart problems. Something more was involved than attitude. Then in the 1980s, Dr. Randolph showed that both heart problems and an overstimulated personality could be brought about by a hypersensitive immune system. More specifically, food and chemical intolerance could cause changes in personality and physical symptoms. The tendency to feel time pressure and multitask occurs at levels I and II stimulus. At this stage, a person feels compelled to work fast and do several things at one time. This often causes the feeling of being overstressed.

Paying attention becomes a problem at level II stimulus when children have ADD and ADHD. Attention Deficit Hyperactivity Disorder occurs in both children and adults. As a special education teacher, I am certainly familiar with this problem. It is a very real problem and not just high-spirited, normal boys who are bored with school. When people hear the term Attention Deficit, they think it means that a child can't pay attention, but that isn't the real problem. The real problem is that he can't choose what he pays attention to. Suppose the teacher is giving directions. Bobby means to pay attention, but then he notices that a man is mowing the lawn outside the classroom window. All of his attention is drawn to the man mowing the lawn. He becomes oblivious to what is happening in the classroom. When the teacher calls his name, he jerks back to reality, but now he has lost the sense of what the teacher is talking about. Then Bobby notices that the teacher aide is using flash cards with a girl at the side of the room. His attention is caught by the way the aide's hands move as she flips the cards. Now Bobby has a blank piece of paper in front of him and doesn't know what to do.

Students at this stage are very easily bored, and they may focus on one or two areas, such as video games, cartoons, baseball statistics, or what the other students are doing. They may seem very clever in these areas, but history, science, and math are boring to them. The teacher can pull together interesting examples, draw on the board, and tell jokes, but their minds simply don't focus on what she is saying. They can't stand to be *bored*. They would rather do something bad to stir things up than be bored.

Teachers sometimes try to isolate ADHD students so that they won't be distracted. Sometimes a type of learning cubical is used. This method usually fails because most of these children hate to be isolated. They can always peek around the edge of the cubical. Their attention can still be captured by a fly on the window or the odd shape of a water stain on the ceiling. I used learning games and activities to capture their attention. Everything from Four Straight to Money Tree made learning fun.

There are adults at level II stimulus who are easily distracted and have real difficulty setting priorities. They tend to become absorbed in unimportant tasks that grab their attention rather than sticking to the real job that needs to be accomplished. Let's say that a husband and wife have sold their house and need to move out in 30 days. The wife asks her husband to clean up the huge stacks of newspapers, magazines, and other clutter that have accumulated in his office. Her husband has every intention of doing it, but on his way to the garage to get a box, he notices that the garage light is flickering. Even though the house has already been sold, and the light is not important, the flicker annoys him, and he has to fix it. He drives to two hardware stores to get parts and then repairs the light fixture. When he gets back to his office, he realizes that he hasn't checked his email. Three hours later his wife finds him still deeply absorbed in his email. Then the mail comes. Right on top is his favorite catalog of remaindered books. He carefully goes through the whole catalog page by page highlighting the books he wants to buy. Finally, he looks at the mail again and notices that one of the stamps did not get cancelled. His wife finds him in the kitchen looking for a saucer so that he can soak the stamp off the envelope. This man has been busy all day. Now he is too tired to face the clutter in his office and there is one day less before they have to be out of the house.

Moving up the stimulus side to stimulus level IV, children with autism focus so intently that they can't pull their mind away from whatever has caught their attention. They can watch a ceiling fan go around or spin the wheels of a toy truck for hours. Temple Grandin writes that as a child she could sit for hours at the beach watching sand dribble through her fingers. She would study each individual grain of sand like a scientist looking through a microscope. As she studied the shapes and colors, she would go into a trance that cut her off from the world around her.[63]

The kinds of games and activities that I used for children with ADHD would not be appropriate for most autistic students. Children with autism need a calm, structured environment with very little visual or auditory stimulation. Temple Grandin tells us how in school she would tune out, shut off her ears, and daydream. Her daydreams would be like Technicolor movies in her head. She could also become completely absorbed in spinning a penny or examining the wood-grain pattern on her desk. Her speech teacher would gently hold her chin to pull her back into the real world.[64]

At level III, when most symptoms become mental rather than physical, people tend to become intensely absorbed in the ideas or causes they become involved in. They do not use what an older generation would call common sense or moderation. Instead, each thing must be carried to the extreme. They are even willing to sacrifice themselves or their own interests. At level III withdrawal, some become vegetarians because of their affinity for animals. They are not satisfied with the practical, commonsense kind of vegetarianism that includes eggs, some dairy, and perhaps fish. No, they must go all the way and become vegans. In addition to not eating meat, fish, or poultry, vegans do not use other animal products such as eggs, dairy products, honey, leather, fur, silk, and wool. Cosmetics and soaps made from animal products are not used.[65] That this is a lot of trouble for their families or that it has possible health consequences does not compute because, in their minds, it is so intensely important for them to be vegans. Some vegans are not satisfied until they become even more extreme or pure. There are the fruitarians and the breatharians: people who actually don't believe humans need to eat.[66]

Many people are becoming involved in protecting our environment. Some people within this group are at level III withdrawal. These people can't moderate their views or accommodate the needs of the rest of the community. If their attention is captured by the need to preserve the pristine wilderness in Alaska, then it becomes intensely important to preserve the entire wilderness. The fact that the security interests of their own nation requires drilling for oil in one small corner of this wilderness is not important because they are willing to sacrifice their own interest or that of their country for the sake of their cause. If they latch onto the idea of saving energy by using fluorescent lights, then they not only exaggerate the amount of energy and money that will be saved, they demand that the government pass a law to force everyone to use fluorescent lights. The fact that disposing of the new light bulbs may cause mercury contamination or that being exposed to these lights can be painful for an autistic person doesn't penetrate the thinking of people at level III withdrawal.[67] For some of these people, the end justifies the means and nothing is as important as their cause. Their moral imperative justifies manipulating the facts, lying, and using a double standard because achieving their goal will save the earth.

Anxiety is the overriding characteristic of level III withdrawal. A person at this level is full of anxiety. If such a person fastens on a danger such as global warming, her anxiety can balloon out of all proportion to any real danger. In *Plenty* magazine, Liz Galst wrote about her anxiety attacks in an article titled "Global Worrying: 'The environment is in peril and anxiety disorders are on the rise.' What's the connection?" The connection is that there are now many people at level III withdrawal. When they are bombarded with news about threats to our environment and the dangers of global warming, they fasten on these dangers and their anxiety builds and builds. Liz Galst describes anxiety attacks that began as a feeling of unease but over several months grew worse until they morphed into panic attacks. The sight of an idling car sending carbon dioxide into the atmosphere would send her into an "hours-long panic, complete with shaking, the sweats, and staring off into space." Instead of using the elevator, she would walk up eight flights of stairs to her apartment to save electricity. At night, she would lay awake worrying about which disaster would happen first and trying to think of how she personally could prevent the catastrophes. There is a name for this syndrome: "eco-anxiety" which is a chronic fear of the environmental future.[68]

Voting patterns may be influenced by whether a person is on the withdrawal or stimulus side of his or her immune system reactions. For example, a person with eco-anxiety (more women than men) will favor a strong government that can protect the environment and provide a large safety net. Those on the stimulus side (more men than women) will want a small government and more individual freedom.

Continuing down the withdrawal side, an Alzheimer's patient at level IV withdrawal may become quite determined to do something that really isn't in her own best interest, which is especially true in the early stages of the disease. This can drive her family crazy. She may be determined to change her will. Even though she forgets everything else, she won't forget the idea of the will. Once her attention has been focused on the will, she won't drop it. It may not be the will. It may be that she wants to give an expensive gift to each of her grandchildren even though that is beyond her means. It could be that she is determined to visit her old friend. No matter how many times her daughter explains that the friend lives in another state, she is sure that the friend lives just on the other side of the hill. She opens the door and starts walking to her friend's house. Let us assume that her daughter sees her and brings her back. She may have to bring her mother back many times. It is surprising that even with Alzheimer's disease, in which the defining characteristic is loss of memory, there is still a tendency to fasten determinedly to an idea and hang on to it.

Under "Attention," we have looked at everything from multitasking to autism to "tunnel vision." There is only space left at the top of the stimulus scale. At this level, there are more and more young people, usually young men, who are focused on just one thing or a few subjects that interest them. Their minds are so stimulated that they are highly intelligent, but they have trouble relating to other people and the rest of life. Some are hooked on video games. They resent being pulled away from their games and are bored by other activities. Geeks are known for their obsessive interest in obscure topics. It is almost as if the mind likes to amuse itself by thinking of all kinds of questions and answers on a subject that doesn't really matter. On www.gibberish.com, one self-described geek wrote about his fascination with the way burritos are folded. A taqueria-style burrito is steamed until the edges are almost sealed. Then it is wrapped in foil almost like a candy bar. Other burritos are left open-ended and don't have foil and on and on. His friend finally told him that it might be better if he spent a lot less time thinking about burritos.

Sometimes this tendency to be obsessive is put to good use in a career. It may be the key to success for someone such as an investor or a program developer. Sebastian

Mallaby, author of *More Money than God*, a fascinating book about the hedge fund industry, was interviewed on CSPAN. Since Mallaby was clearly comfortable dealing with the intricate details of this complex industry, he was asked if he would like to help manage a hedge fund. Mallaby explained that to make money in a hedge fund you have to be so focused that it becomes an obsession. You have to be addicted to watching your stock positions minute by minute. He enjoys telling stories and would rather write books.[69]

Others spend hours on the Internet. Hackers delight in unraveling computer codes and playing with their techie toys. Many hackers love to stoke up on caffeine and sugar (and probably pizza and other foods they are reacting to) for all-night hacking sessions. The most successful ones are able to upload vast amounts of seemingly meaningless data into their memories that can be used later to unravel computer programs. Eric Raymond, author of the New Hacker's Dictionary, mentions learning the complex typesetting language needed for the first version of his book in about four workdays by virtually "inhaling" the 477 page Knuth's manual. He was surprised at his editor's "flabbergasted reaction" because this ability was considered routine among his hacker friends.[70]

Despite the almost superhuman abilities of some people at level III stimulus to memorize data and manipulate the ideas that hold their attention, they are bored by the mundane needs of everyday life. Hackers often don't bother to pay their bills on time and an unbelievable amount of clutter builds up. It is only the thing that has grabbed their attention that matters.

At the extreme end of level III and IV stimulus are the mass murderers and the serial killers. The motivations of these two types are very different. If a mass murderer walks into a restaurant, shoots six strangers, and kills himself, the police expect to find a social isolate. Detectives are not surprised when neighbors say that the killer stayed in his apartment and never talked with anyone. This would be the man who is so stimulated that he has lost any compassion or emotional connectedness to other people and resents any real or imagined slight that has been done to him. Perhaps he thinks his boss does not appreciate how brilliant he is, or maybe he thinks that his girlfriend has laughed about him behind his back. His anger builds as he goes over and over how unfair it is. His attention is focused with laser-like intensity on how he has been wronged. Getting revenge becomes the only thing that matters. Even if he has to sacrifice himself, he must do it.

There is another type of mass murderer who is harder to understand. This is the young man who is friendly and well liked, yet will walk into a classroom and shoot a dozen students at random before he shoots himself.

This is the man who is at level III withdrawal where the symptoms are primarily mental rather than physical. However, he is still on the withdrawal side. People at level III withdrawal are known for their sweetness. They are unusually nice because they are not aggressive and hate violence. They often have problems with anxiety and depression, but they may be passionately involved in a cause that has captured their attention. Suppose such a man begins to obsess about his personal problems or the justice of his cause. He can flip from the withdrawal side to level III stimulus. Then he becomes secretive, determined, and violent. What can trigger such a change? It could be reactions to medication or suddenly stopping medication. It could also be triggered by chemical and food intolerance.

The "timid" friend whom I wrote about earlier told me of an experience that helps to illustrate this type of reaction. She was afraid of her husband and easily intimidated by him, but after one chemical reaction, she wanted to kill him. Her husband kept a can of solvent in the car that was used to clean the engine. The lid did not fit tightly. The can tipped over and the solvent seeped into the back of the car as he drove 50 miles across the desert. The next morning, she opened the car door and was hit in the face with the fumes. She ran to the house, crying and screaming, "What did you do to the car?" She said that she actually saw red and wanted to get a gun and kill her husband. It took her 10 to 15 minutes to calm down. She also said that she had this rage response one other time after walking into a building where herbicide had just been used.

Serial killers are out for their own gratification. Sexual desires and the lust for power have gotten mixed up with their intensely overstimulated personalities. They care about only one thing, and with their truncated emotions, they have no remorse for the terrible things they have done. Unlike mass murderers, serial killers usually do not kill themselves when capture is near.

Perhaps if I had not worked for years with children who had attention deficit disorder, I would not have thought about the role that attention plays in our personalities. If we can't focus or pay attention, we can't learn. If we can't control what we focus on, or if we focus too intently on one thing, our personalities can be disturbed. At each level of food and chemical intolerance, our ability to pay attention is affected.

CONNECTEDNESS

WE ARE BECOMING LESS AND LESS CONNECTED to our group, our culture, our friends, and our family. Dr. Weston Price was deeply moved when he saw the Swiss of the Loetschental Valley observe their national holiday:

> If one is fortunate enough to be in the valley in early August and witness the earnestness with which the people celebrate their national holiday, he will be privileged to see a sight long to be remembered. These celebrations close with the gathering together of the mountaineers on various crags and prominences where great bonfires are lighted from fuel that has been accumulated and built into an enormous mound to make a huge torchlight. These bonfires are lighted at a given hour from end to end of the valley throughout its expanse. Every mountaineer on a distant crag seeing the lights knows that the others are signaling to him that they, too, are making their sacred consecration in song, which says "one for all and all for one." This motive has been crystallized

into action and has become a part of the very souls of the people. One understands why doors do not need to be bolted in the Loetschental Valley.[71]

Our own national holidays no longer seem to reach our hearts. We go through the motions. The audience on the Fourth of July is filled with the gray heads of what is left of the World War II generation. Even Christmas is slipping away. First, it was trivialized by Santa Claus and plastic toys, and now it is being pushed aside by Winter Break. Those of us with treasured memories of opening gifts with our family on Christmas morning, and perhaps a nativity program or candle-light service at church, feel a sadness deep inside at what is being lost. We usually blame atheists and political activists with no sense of history or common sense for stealing our traditions. However, there is a more basic problem. People on the stimulus side easily become bored by family traditions. As each generation becomes weaker, fewer and fewer people really love and care about their heritage.

Drs. Friedman and Rosenman saw this happening 40 years ago. They observed that those with an overstimulated behavior pattern might still go to traditional gatherings such as Thanksgiving, but they were inwardly annoyed and irritated. These people felt they were wasting their time and accomplishing very little. The more bored and irritated they were, the more disconnected they were.[72]

True friendship has also been disappearing at level I and II stimulus. It is not that these people don't have friends; it is that they have many friends that don't mean very much to them. Friedman and Rosenman observed that many of their heart patients who had Type A Personality had many acquaintances, but hardly anyone who was really close to them. They might have scores, even hundreds of acquaintances, but they were almost all business contacts. They prided themselves on their network of friends. In fact, they were focused on business and conversation that didn't involve their business tended to bore them.[73]

Social networking now enables us to have thousands of friends, but in what sense are these friends? This gives us the illusion of having lots of friends. As Daniel Goleman writes in *Social Intelligence,* "Technology offers more varieties of nominal communication in actual isolation."[74]

Something unexpected happens to our connection to other human beings at level III withdrawal. People begin to care more and more about animals until some care more about animals than they do about people. Looking back about 15 years, to the time that I was still quite ill with environmental illness, I can see that this was happening to me. Mother and I and our beautiful German shepherd, Susie, were living right on the Mexican border, in Jacumba, California. One afternoon, Susie nipped a teenage boy, and later she was quarantined. I was more anxious and upset than I let people see. I was afraid that she could be put down if there was another incident. I was determined to protect my dog no matter what the cost. I fantasized about sneaking her over the border into Mexico or moving to another state. In reality, all I did was watch her like a hawk and keep her on a leash, but my feelings were so intense that I might have done something really foolish.

Healthy people tend to be quite practical about animals. After all, throughout the centuries most people have lived on farms and raised animals for food. By the time I retired, my immune system problem was much better. I got an adorable little corgi. Somehow, I didn't bond with him as I had with my German shepherds. Then I learned that I needed cancer surgery and would be away from home. My new dog just wasn't working out. The sister of a friend was eager to have a corgi. I was very practical about the whole thing and gave her the dog.

Shortly before I retired, I had my house appraised. This was in the midst of the real estate boom, and I got a much better estimate than I had expected. A neighbor asked me over to see what I thought his house might be worth. As I walked in, he laughingly told me that he would never get married again unless he needed his wife's money to pay the mortgage. We walked through the house. There were pictures of jungle animals in the living room. The extra bedroom was filled with exercise equipment, but he was going to get rid of it. He was no longer interested in bodybuilding. He had lost weight and had taken on the look of a typical thin, level III withdrawal person. When we walked into his bedroom, I saw that it was decorated with large pictures of wolves! He had probably lost his closeness to his wife before their divorce, and he was probably becoming more and more connected to animals.

A dear friend has been looking forward to retiring with her husband of many years. She recently confided to me, "He cares more about the dogs than he does about me."

Alzheimer's patients often become very anxious about their pets. One friend told me that his 88-year-old mother had often called him at work because she was so worried about what would happen to her gray cat, Crissey, when she died. His mother would be in tears because she was so upset. Finally, he gave her a beautiful birthday card with a picture of a large cat on the front. Inside he wrote a loving note promising to take care of Crissey if anything happened to her. The card was taped near her wheelchair. When she got anxious, she could look at the card and be reassured.

Most people at level III withdrawal care deeply about animals. They can pour out their love to a pet in a way that they can't show love to another person. They may spend an inordinate amount of time rescuing stray dogs and cats or trying to save injured animals. A large number of people at level III withdrawal become vegetarians or near vegetarians because they can't bear to hurt or kill animals. The cover of *E: The Environmental Magazine* featured the face of a large gorilla behind bars with the title of the lead article: "OUR **AGONY** OVER ANIMALS: Achieving Empathy for the Non-Human World is a Slow and Painful Process." The word *agony* was highlighted in deep red.

There are things besides animals that people become attached to. Some care more about things. This takes an odd twist in the hoard and clutter syndrome, packrat syndrome, or compulsive hoarding. People save more and more things and are not able to give them up. This happens most often at level II and III withdrawal when people are low in energy and have trouble making decisions. They don't seem to have the energy to do what it takes to stay organized and get rid of things. However, it is not just a matter of energy. They will go to endless trouble to clip articles and file them or sort things from one pile to another. They may even mail information to a friend or donate clothing. The thing they can't do is to just throw something away.

Junk mail has been a disaster for people with this compulsion. There is an article on cancer that should be sent to a friend and another one on diabetes that would be really important for another friend. Several catalogs have excellent bargains on warm winter clothing, and there is some really significant political analysis that a person doesn't want to lose. All of this stuff has to be saved. There is more the next day and the next day. Sunday is the only day that the junk mail doesn't come, and there is twice as much mail on Monday! The junk mail is added to all the other old things that can't be thrown away, and the clutter grows. Some people become embarrassed to have anyone over. Sometimes there is nothing left but narrow paths winding through the stacks of clutter. Some people can't sell their house because they are overwhelmed by the amount of junk that needs to be moved.

Now there are even professional organizers. In walks a slim, bubbly, Type A professional with her baskets and labels. She sets her client to work sorting clutter into baskets labeled "donations," "trash," and "keep." Meanwhile, our expert paints the focal wall red and starts assembling precut, manufactured shelving. She leaves her enthusiastic client with plenty of baskets, all neatly labeled and not a scrap of clutter on any table. Does our professional organizer come back a year later to see if her plan is being followed? Never! Nobody has helped our clutter bug with the underlying health problems that cause her low energy and her difficulty making decisions, so nothing really changes.

I had a pretty good system. I put everything that I might need later in a box without agonizing too long over whether to keep it or not. When the box was full, I put it in the garage. Two or three years later, after everything had become outdated and worthless, I would throw it away. However, there were always stacks of papers on my table and clutter on the kitchen counters. Not long ago, I suddenly realized that I had become a whole new person. I was no longer willing to tolerate the junk. Instead of thinking "oh, well," I thought "it will only take a second." After preparing lunch, instead of ignoring the mess, I would quickly put a few things away and have a beautiful clean counter. Who would have thought that going off of grain and sugar would help a person become tidy and organized!

Going up the stimulus ladder, possessions can become important in a different way. Personal relationships play only a small part in the lives of people at level III stimulus. They often become deeply involved in a hobby or collection. They may become obsessed with obtaining a certain piece of art. Vacation time may be spent searching for rare books while other family members stay at home. Money, which is needed by the family, may go into the purchase of a painting or an exquisite piece of antique jewelry.

After I moved back to the Northwest, a friend I had known in school years ago invited me over. She had to be my age, but she seemed much younger. She was slim, stylish, and energetic. Her home was modest but beautifully decorated. The walls were covered with paintings. She told me, "My life is art." She explained in detail how she had obtained individual paintings. Some had been quite costly while talented friends had given her others. There was no clutter on the tables. She had the energy to keep everything orderly. We didn't see very much of her husband. He had quickly retreated to his office. His space was a rather dark, cluttered room at the back of the house. She had taken over all the rest of the house, and she was annoyed with him for not straightening his area. Visiting this very superior, level III stimulus woman made me so glad to get home.

We will conclude the illustrations of connectedness at the different stages of food and chemical intolerance with autism on the stimulus side. Children with autism are not able to connect with the emotions of others. They actually feel more comfortable playing with robots than with other human children. Robots are humanoid without human emotions. Eye tracking research has shown autistic children prefer looking at objects rather than human faces. They have difficulty understanding facial expressions.[75] Kaspar is a friendly robot from England. He has been programmed to do things like smile, frown, laugh, blink, and wave he arms. One mother said that before her daughter played with Kaspar, she would make a smiley face no matter what emotion you asked her to make. After playing with Kaspar, the daughter started to put the right emotion with the right face. Another little girl, Eden, used to recoil when other girls held her hand and turned stiff if they tried to cuddle her. After playing with the robot, she became a lot more affectionate. Now she hugs everyone.[76][77]

Bandit is an endearing little robot from the University of Southern California. He has cartoon-like features, which are easy for children to interpret. Playing with Bandit seems to increase social interaction.[78]

The most advanced robot for autistic children is Zeno, a 27-inch, life-like, talking robot developed by Hanson Robokind in Arlington Texas. The robot's soft, flexible, life-like skin enables him to smile, frown, and even show disappointment. A lot of the therapies for autistic children involve mimicking appropriate behavior. The robot might say to the child, "Tell me when you think I'm happy, or sad, or when I'm mad at you." The success of the therapy is based on the ability of the robot to have expressions. Fred Margolin, Hanson Robokind CEO, tells of taking Zeno to the Autism Treatment Center of Dallas:

> We took the robot over to work with two mid to lower spectrum kids who had not been talking whatsoever to staff, and in ten minutes, the kids started talking to the robots. The staff was teared up and crying.

Zeno is expected to be available to the public in the summer of 2012 at a cost of $3,000 to $5,000.[79] This is one bright spot in a tragic story. When I started writing this book, people were saying that 1 out of every 127 children had autism. Now the figure is 1 out of 88.

SELF-CONTROL

I HAD BEEN DOING VERY WELL ON MY DIET. IT seemed easy to stick to it. Then I went to lunch with a friend and ate some things I shouldn't. Later that afternoon, when the food reactions kicked in, I just wanted to go off my diet a little bit. Just some butter on my sprouted grain roll. Oh, that tasted so good. Well a little peanut butter wouldn't be too bad. You know how this story goes. That is not the part that surprised me. What surprised me was that I didn't want to do anything that was good for me. It was time to take some vitamins. No, I didn't want to swallow any pills. I should do the exercises I had skipped. No, I didn't want to exercise. I didn't want to do anything good. I wanted to do something bad. (That might mean ice cream, but it could mean sitting like a lump in front of the TV or going shopping.)

Most of our population born after 1960 is living from one fix to the next, whether it is cake and cookies, bread and cereal, ice cream and milk, coffee and chocolate, cell phones and tech toys, or candles and air fresheners. Not only do they not want to give up their addictions, but many of them don't want to do anything that is good for them. At level I stimulus, people are trim, energetic, and in top form. However, they often seem out-of-control and immature. They want what they want when they want it. They love their fast food and diet soft drinks. Their energy is fueled by the lift they get from the foods and chemicals that they are reacting to. If they wait too long for the next shot of fructose, aspartame, wheat gluten, or whatever they are reacting to, they begin to feel a little down or tired.

At the grocery store, several attractive, Type A, young people were buying things for a fun dinner. They were calling to each other so everyone could hear them. They were getting chips, dips, ice cream, and other things that weren't good for them. It sounded as though this wasn't their usual diet, but for this occasion, they were determined to have junk food. One young man said in high glee that this would really be a "bad dinner." When you are addicted, bad is good, and you celebrate your indulgences. "Comfort food" is the answer to stress, and advertisers encourage us to have a "me moment" or a "mini escape."

It is at level II stimulus that the lack of self-control starts becoming a real problem. Children with learning problems don't just have attention problems, but they also have poor impulse control. A student with ADHD may suddenly get out of his chair and walk around the room, speak out loudly, or kick someone under the table without any regard to the class rules or the need to maintain a calm learning environment. With his lack of self-discipline and his difficulty focusing on schoolwork, very little homework is turned in.

Poor impulse control leads to difficulty with delayed gratification. I gave out "tickets" to reward good work and behavior. This immediate reward worked very well. Every Friday we counted our tickets. The children loved to count their tickets and save them. Five times a year we had Prize Day. My students were very generous about using their tickets to get gifts for their brothers, sisters, mothers, and fathers. I planned one Prize Day right before Christmas Vacation so that they could use the gifts for Christmas and save their families a little money. However, most of them couldn't wait that long. They gave their gifts as soon as they got home and then begged their parents to take them to the mall and get more gifts for Christmas!

My grandmother was a wonderful, warm, loving person. Looking back, I realize that she was a level II person. When we visited Grandmother, the breakfast table was loaded with all the comfort food that she and I both loved. There were stacks of buttered toast, platters of bacon, plates of bear-claw coffeecake, tall glasses of milk, and fresh squeezed orange juice. Mother didn't let us eat like that at home. One thing we knew about Grandmother, she couldn't keep a secret. She didn't have the impulse control. She just had to tell!

Weight problems catch up with us at level II stimulus. If you have ever had a weight problem, you know how food reactions can destroy your self-control. You can be so good all day and then in the evening you just can't seem to stop eating. You eat all of the things that you have been denying yourself and more than make up for the calories that you saved at breakfast and lunch. You kick yourself. You blame yourself. You think that your weight problems are all your own fault for being so weak. Overeating is a symptom, not the cause, of your problems. Your underlying problem is your intolerance to certain foods and chemicals.

This is the way it works. You have cornflakes with milk for breakfast, and it tastes good and you feel satisfied. You are reacting to corn, but the reaction doesn't set in for several hours. By lunch, you need more corn to keep going. You microwave a Mexican frozen dinner for lunch. Both meals are low in calories. You congratulate yourself on how well you are doing on your diet. By the time you get home from work, the reactions are really setting in. Sometimes they are low blood sugar reactions. Your body knows how to get what it wants. Your self-control slinks away. Now you not only want corn, you want something sweet, and you can't seem to stop snacking.

Some dieters have tried to tell nutritionists that they do better when they skip breakfast. Nutritionists will have none of that. They insist that breakfast is the most important meal of the day. This is no doubt true for a healthy person without food intolerance. What the dieter has discovered is that the later in the day she eats, the longer she can avoid the reactions and the cravings that do her in. The trouble is that when she does eat, she will probably eat something she is reacting to and be trapped again.

There is an element of compulsion to the food cravings that we feel. Food cravings are not the same thing as hunger. It is not that we are hungry and any food, whether it is safe food or food you are craving, will fill us up and satisfy us. Your body wants what it is reacting to. Let's say that you come home from work and you feel like having cheese crackers. You have decided that you are not going to eat any more of those cheese crackers (but you know there is a box up in the cupboard), so you decide to have roast and leftover potato salad instead. You eat quite a bit because you are trying to get full. You still aren't satisfied, so you eat ice cream, and then some cookies, and finally the cheese crackers. Some writers of diet books have even suggested that you should just go ahead and eat the cheese crackers to begin with and save yourself all the extra calories that you consume trying to avoid them.

Most dieters have learned that they can't take the first one. If they are serious about not eating the cookies at Mom's house, they must not eat the first cookie. Eating the first one destroys their will power. Alcoholics have also learned that they can't take the first drink. Both obesity and alcoholism occur at level II stimulus. In fact, Dr. Randolph does not distinguish between food addiction and alcohol addiction. He found that an alcoholic isn't just reacting to alcohol. Such a person is really reacting to the foods that his favorite drinks are made from such as corn and yeast. Those who are intolerant of wheat typically react to roasted barley or malt. Dr. Randolph called alcoholism the "acme of the food-allergy problem" because alcohol is absorbed more rapidly than food. It is absorbed all along the gastrointestinal tract, including the mouth, the stomach, and the intestines. Food is mainly absorbed in the intestines. This means that a person can get a faster and more intense high from the alcoholic form of a food. Suppose that a person who is reacting to corn abstains from alcohol, but they continue to eat corn. Perhaps he carries a roll of hard candies made from corn syrup in his pocket or keeps some in his desk. He will continue to be plagued by cravings unless he gives up corn completely.[80]

The loss of will power, which occurs at level II stimulus, can open a person to other addictions that don't appear to be related to foods. Suppose a slightly heavy level II stimulus woman eats cheese and crackers for lunch. She knows that she should vacuum the house, but not long after eating, she has an urge to have some fun. She decides to go shopping. She loves to shop. She has promised her husband that she won't use the credit cards, but she does have a little cash in her purse. She wants to do something "bad," just a little bit bad. She stands inside the mall entrance and takes a deep breath. She loves the mall. The chemicals in the air further stimulate her and add to her sense of satisfaction. She is drawn to a store with a large SALE sign. Inside she spots a darling little red dress. Her attention is captured by the special shade of red and the pleats on the bodice of the dress. She loves the red purse and shoes that are displayed with the dress. The whole outfit costs much more than the cash she has, but she has to have it. She pulls out her credit cards. Her self-control has long since vanished. She rushes home without trying anything on and puts everything in the back of the closet. The next morning she realizes that the outfit is too small and that she will probably never wear it. She is filled with remorse. This episode didn't start with the SALE sign or the attractive display. It started with the cheese and crackers and the air in the mall. In the same way, gambling addiction can be enhanced by eating foods that a person is reacting to, usually followed by alcohol, and finally stimulated by the air in the casino.

At levels I and II, the issues involve a lack of self-control. Out-of-control food cravings are often obvious, as with the husband who always has to have a huge bowl of ice cream after dinner or the woman who easily puts away two quarts of milk every day. At level III, food sensitivity is not as easy to observe because normal to small amounts of food are often adequate to satisfy a person's cravings. These people tend to graze all day unobtrusively on the foods they are reacting to. At level III, the issue is too much control rather than too little self-control.

Anorexia Nervosa seems to belong to level III withdrawal. This is self-control to the point of death. This disorder is characterized by an extreme fear of getting fat and the relentless pursuit of thinness. Ninety percent of those with anorexia are women. Even though they become emaciated, they think they are too fat. They do not want to be looked at. I suspect that this aversion to being looked at and the idea that they are ugly because they are fat are related to the fear of being looked at discussed earlier in this book. This disorder is usually accompanied by depression and anxiety, the defining characteristics of level III withdrawal.[81]

We can get some idea of what it must be like to be anorexic from an article at www.lifescript.com, "In Her Own Words: Living with Anorexia & Bulimia." At the time that the article was written, Joanne was a dietitian living in Illinois. She had fully recovered from her anorexia. Joanne showed the first signs of anorexia when she was in the tenth grade. She was a synchronized swimmer, and she wanted to look better in a bathing suit. She started by skipping lunch. During lunch period, she would study or talk casually to her friends as if she had already eaten. She often stayed late at school and skipped dinner. She exercised compulsively. Sometimes she even worked out all night. She didn't like to sleep because she would burn fewer calories. When she turned 16, there were more parties and gatherings with friends. If she had to eat something, she would compensate for that by purging and taking pills. She took up to 25 or 30 laxatives, diet pills, and water pills a day.

Joanne says that during this period she was very moody and temperamental. She lost weight. She always felt cold. Sometimes she fainted. Toward the end, fine baby hair grew on her stomach, a common sign of anorexia. The enamel on her teeth eroded, and she needed many fillings due to exposure to stomach acid when she threw up. All the vomiting she did caused her lower esophageal sphincter to loosen, so she still suffers from reflux disease.

Joanne tried to get a fresh start in college. She behaved like a normal freshman and gained 15 pounds. She thought she was ugly and fat. She started to get back into her anorexic habits. This time she wanted to change. She called home and asked her mother to find help. She was not able to enter the first program that was suggested because she was a vegetarian. She did find a psychiatrist that she could empathize with, and he helped her to recover from her anorexia.[82]

Anorexia fits closely into the patterns that would be expected at level III withdrawal. Look first at attention. A woman with anorexia focuses like a laser on one thing—that she is fat and must get thin. This is a distorted view, but a person from the real world can't break through and make her see herself as she really is. She loses her common sense. Her determination to get thin is so intense that she is willing to break the rules. She knows that she shouldn't use laxatives, diet pills, and vomiting, but nothing matters except getting thin. The end justifies the means. Vegetarianism is another thing that we have seen at level III withdrawal. Vegetarianism is quite common among anorexics. Anxiety and depression are often a problem. Add to these traits the fact that many women at level III withdrawal do not like to be looked at. Finally, add a heightened degree of self-control: control to the point of self-destruction.

Anorexia is a very serious condition. It is the leading cause of death among people seeking psychiatric help. Many people have found that food sensitivity is involved in some way. Websites often suggest that scratch tests or the RAST test should be used to uncover allergies. However, these tests often do not expose many of the substances that provoke food and chemical intolerance. It would be better to have thorough testing by a qualified Clinical Ecologist.

Dr. Randolph found that at level III withdrawal, symptoms became mental rather than physical. First among these is anxiety. Add to this difficulty making decisions, poor memory, and depression. A certain softness or sentimentality is also part of the picture. These symptoms help to explain some of the problems that are commonly grouped under OCD, obsessive-compulsive disorder. OCD involves an odd type of control. This is not a lack of self-control or an excess of control, instead it is control from within a person that makes him do things he doesn't want to do! The first two types, the checkers and the hoarders, can be explained by typical level III withdrawal traits.

One large group with OCD is said to be the "checkers." These people perform excessive checking rituals. Before leaving home, a checker might have to check the gas, check the oven, the windows, the door locks, the basement, and the pet door. Then, half way to work she might start worrying about whether she really checked the oven. She becomes very anxious about what could happen if the oven has been left on. She returns home to double check the oven and has to double-check everything else before she can start to work again. I can tell you from my own experience that this need to check stems from poor memory combined with anxiety over what will happen if you don't make sure by going back and checking.

Suppose you are paying a bill by mail. You seal the envelope. Then you realize that you might have put the wrong bill in the envelope. Then you wonder if you put the check in. Finally, you have to be sure that you signed the check. Each time you have to open the envelope and pull everything out so that you can check. Someone observing this behavior might think it was a ritual, but you can't actually remember and you need to be sure. You don't want to admit that your memory is that bad because it is too close to Alzheimer's for comfort. When I got off of most of the foods and chemicals that I was reacting to, my memory improved and my checking behavior disappeared.

Checking behavior is sometimes combined with other compulsions and becomes quite bizarre. One patient checked every chair for pins or pieces of glass. Another man checked every trash bag as he went by to be sure that it really contained garbage and not a corpse.[83]

Hoarding is another OCD behavior that comes out of the traits that belong to level III withdrawal. Hoarding has already been discussed under "Connectedness" because it involves becoming more attached to things instead of people. Suppose you are not sure which receipts you need to keep, but you are filled with anxiety over having adequate records in case you need them. Wouldn't it be best just to keep any kind of record? Suppose you are attached to all the little things your children used to play with and couldn't possibly give up the things that belonged to your mother. You save newspapers and health newsletters that might be important to your friends, and of course, you have to save any catalogs that you might use later. Soon there are piles and piles of stuff. You are filled with anxiety at the thought of losing any of it, and you can't decide what to throw away. Clutter at level II withdrawal is primarily about low energy, but hoarding at level III withdrawal is primarily about anxiety and the inability to make decisions.

Chemical sensitivity plays a major role in hoarding. People at level III withdrawal often have serious reactions to chemicals that can be tolerated by most people. Reactions to the chemicals in paper and print are very common. Imagine what happens when a person with this problem starts sorting junk mail. As she reads and handles the mail, she breathes in chemicals and touches the ink. Colored pictures in magazines are especially bad, and scented inserts are disastrous. She loves to read just as a milk addict loves milk. She doesn't realize that her mind is being affected, but she becomes confused and can't seem to throw anything away. Her ability to make a decision is practically paralyzed. As the junk piles up in her house, the chemicals also build up and she may become increasingly odd.

What I think of as "real" OCD involves unwanted thoughts or feelings that must be appeased with special actions or rituals. Obsessions are baseless, persistent, and disturbing thoughts that are uncontrollable and unstoppable. They repeat endlessly and a person can't get them out of his head. A person realizes that these upsetting thoughts are not based on reality and are coming from his own mind. He usually tries to fight against them or get rid of them, but the ideas or images keep coming back.

Compulsions are repetitive behaviors or rituals that are carried out to relieve the worry and tension caused by the obsessions. These behaviors appear to be senseless, excessive, and unreasonable. Sometimes compulsive behavior is not directly related to an obsession but must be done for things to "feel right." For example, one young woman was sure that she would become "fat" or a "bad person" if she wore blue. She spent hours choosing things to wear that didn't have any blue in them. She checked over and over for blue specks or threads. She also walked through doorways a "right" number of times. Some people must do things over and over until they feel right. One young man also had to go through doorways over and over until he felt just right. He had to get in and out of bed over and over as well. He always had to step on the carpet with his left foot first, and he climbed the stairs sideways.[84] A newly married woman began to avoid the number four. She was afraid that something dreadful would happen to her husband if she used that number.

His birthday was on the fourth day of the month. She would skip the fourth page of books she was reading. She never wrote the number four. She would never eat four of anything and on and on. Gradually the compulsion spread to include numbers beginning or ending with four, multiples of four, and the numbers adjacent to four. That is when she finally got help.[85]

It has been noted that many people with OCD tend to have an exaggerated idea of the danger that they or a loved one is faced with. They also have an exaggerated sense of being personally responsible for preventing the disaster.[86] For example, a woman may feel that if she does not get clean enough after she goes to the bathroom, she might touch someone and cause him to get a terrible disease. She washes and washes until her hands and arms are red and raw, but she can't seem to get clean enough. Her real fear is not for herself. It is really a fear of being responsible for harming someone else. A little girl may have a feeling of doom that her father is going to die in a plane crash. When he is gone, she might develop a ritual of touching the walls in her bedroom without stepping on the rug. This must be done three times a day, precisely the same way every time. If she is interrupted, or if she makes a mistake, the whole ritual must be repeated. She has a terrible feeling that if she doesn't do this exactly right her father will die.

A person with OCD has insight into his or her problem. He or she knows that his or her obsessions come from his or her own mind and are not really valid. They even realize that their compulsive behavior is irrational. He or she even realizes that his or her compulsive behavior is irrational. This contrasts with schizophrenia in which a patient really believes that there are devils sitting on the tree limb laughing at him.[87] However, even though he or she knows it is irrational, he or she must complete his or her ritualistic compulsions.

OCD is classified as an anxiety disorder. Remember that anxiety and depression are the hallmarks of level III withdrawal. The possibility that this behavior is caused by food and chemical intolerance should be investigated. The roasted sunflower seeds that she is always munching, the gas stove in the kitchen, or the scented deodorant that she wears could all cause this behavior. Careful testing for food and chemical intolerance should be one of the alternatives that a family considers.

We blame ourselves if we don't have enough self-control. Friends and family are mystified if a person is so determined to reach a goal, such as getting thin, that he or she will actually harm themselves. Either too little or too much self-control can be a sign that a person is reacting to foods and chemicals. Identifying and eliminating possible allergens should be explored.

CONFLICT

THERE IS A CONTINUUM OF AGGRESSION THAT moves from passivity, acceptance, and appeasement to assertiveness, irritability, aggravation, anger, rage, and violence. The early stages of assertion may be beneficial to an individual and even to society, but we are seeing more and more cases of unprovoked rage and violence. We are also seeing an increase in individuals with diminished emotions who can't handle conflict. Where do these feelings come from? Are the causes psychological or are there underlying biological reasons?

Surprising clues can be found in the drawings of young children when they are being tested for allergies. Doris Rapp, M.D. is a well-known clinical ecologist and pediatrician whose expertise I will be relying on heavily in the chapter on testing for allergies. When Dr. Rapp does provocation/neutralization (P/N) allergy testing, she usually has the child write his name while he or she is being tested. Sometimes she has the child draw a picture or color a picture from a coloring book. This reveals changes in mood and coordination brought on by the food or chemical being tested. Adults are usually able to avoid exposing their emotions, but the anger and hostility in some allergic children can be clearly demonstrated by the pictures that they draw when they react to specific allergy extracts.

Prior to being tested for oranges, Andy played nicely with the other children in the testing room, but after the orange extract was administered, he became aggressive. He pinched his mother, broke his pencils, and acted very upset and angry. He drew a stick figure of his mom hanging from a yardarm and then another stick figure labeled "mom" that was full of bullet holes. Under the stick figures was a tombstone with the words R.I.P. DEAD MOM. He printed his name with large, bold, poorly coordinated letters. After the neutralization dose for orange was given, Andy neatly printed his name and drew a calm, neutral looking stick figure. After the testing, it was clear why he had been obnoxious, disobedient, and abusive at home after he had orange juice for breakfast.[88]

When Gary, a twelve-year-old boy, was tested for milk, he became silly and talkative. He also became congested and started coughing. Then he became aggressive and drew an angry picture of a shark eating a large creature. He called the picture "Sharkopolis." After he received his neutralization dose, he was pleasant again and felt fine.[89]

During testing for mold, Shawn became sad and angry. This seven-year-old drew a face similar to the draw-a-man pictures that kindergarten teachers ask their students to produce. Shawn's drawing had two eyes, a nose, a line for the mouth, a squiggle of hair, and even two little circles for ears. The difference was that the face drawn before the mold test had a pleasant upturned mouth while the mouth drawn during the test turned down sharply in a harsh line. During the test, Shawn became uncooperative and hostile. He said that he hated his nurse. After the neutralization dose, Shawn drew a happy face and said that he liked his nurse again.[90]

The impact of these drawings is almost shocking when you see the actual art. These drawings and many others are reproduced in Dr. Rapp's books *Is This Your Child?* and *Is This Your Child's World?* Dr. Rapp was well aware of the significance of the changing emotions that she repeatedly witnessed when testing children for allergies. As she said, "Might such reactions help explain some of the unprovoked aggression so pervasive in today's society? This possibility needs intensive, unbiased study."[91]

Sudden unprovoked aggression in both children and adults can be related to allergies and food intolerance. These reactions are frequently associated with red earlobes, restless legs, dark eye circles, and a special "look." Mother's sometimes describe this look in their children as almost demonic. Some children hit, bite kick, spit, and punch when they have been exposed to the wrong food or chemical.[92]

Large, bold, obviously hostile handwriting usually accompanies aggressive stimulus reactions during allergy testing. The handwriting is poorly coordinated and may dissolve into an unintelligible scribble. Children who react on the withdrawal side display a very different type of writing. They write with cramped, teeny, tiny letters, or they may refuse to write. They draw tears, down turned mouths, and other signs of sadness.[93]

Children who react on the withdrawal side will become moody and depressed. They may become unhappy and begin to cry. Some will even curl into a fetal position and jerk away if anyone tries to touch them. A few cower in dark corners or try to hide behind chairs. One teen being tested for ragweed even crawled into the clinic bathtub and refused to come out. After the correct neutralization dose is given, patients quickly return to their normal, pleasant dispositions. Dr. Rapp has videotaped many of these reactions.[94]

When eleven-year-old Marsha was tested with an extract made from the air in her classroom, she curled up and said her head hurt. Her handwriting became very tiny and illegible. Her pulse increased a significant 28 points. She became uncommunicative and threw away her drawing. Ten minutes after the neutralization dose, Marsha said her head was okay and she wanted to draw again.[95] An elimination diet was used to uncover four-year-old Kari's reactions. When she was tested for potatoes, there was a total personality change. She hid in a corner and could not be held, touched, or consoled.[96]

Dr. Rapp was concerned about the quiet children who may never get help with their allergies. Everyone tries to find why a nasty, aggressive child is acting out, but the excessively quiet, shy, irritable, tired, or placid child may never get help with his or her reactions to foods and chemicals.[97]

What happens on the withdrawal side? People at level III withdrawal are the polar opposite of the competitive, aggressive, self-centered Type A personality on the stimulus side. At level III withdrawal, these people can't handle conflict. An argument or an emotional upset in the family will leave them drained and depressed. When they react to foods and chemicals in the environment instead of having a physical symptom such as a headache or arthritis, it is their mind and mood that are affected. They feel helpless and anxious. This is the peacemaker who will appease the aggressive child or the demanding husband.

Research on the personalities of cancer patients can help us understand the characteristics of people on the withdrawal side. In 1979, Richard Sagebiel, M.D., head of the Melanoma Clinic at the University of California San Francisco, noticed a pattern of personality traits in his melanoma patients. He invited Lydia Temoshok, PhD., a nationally recognized researcher in the area of behavioral medicine, to study his patients. When Dr. Temoshok interviewed 150 of these patients, she found strikingly similar characteristics. Seventy-five percent of these melanoma patients were "overwhelmingly nice." They were exceedingly nice, uncomplaining, and unassertive.[98] According to Dr. Temoshok:

1. They were patient, unassertive, cooperative, and appeasing with family, friends, and colleagues at work. They were also accepting of external authority.

2. They did not express emotions and were often unaware of any feelings of anger, past or present.

3. They tended to not experience or express any other negative emotions such as fear, anxiety, or sadness.

4. They were overly worried about meeting other's needs and insufficiently concerned with meeting their own needs. They were often extremely self-sacrificing.

5. They were "notoriously prone to guilt and self-blame."[99]

Dr. Temoshok identified this cluster of traits as the "Type C" personality. "C" is for cancer. She also observed and verified a correlation between the amount of apparent emotional repression in a patient and the progress of their cancer. Patients who were more emotionally expressive had thinner tumors, more slowly dividing cancer cells, and a higher number of immune cells invading the tumor. Patients who were less emotionally expressive had thicker tumors, more rapidly dividing cancer cells, and far fewer immune cells invading the tumor.[100]

What causes this passive personality? The explanation that first occurs to most people is that Type C people are repressing their emotions and this in turn represses the immune system. Therapists have even told cancer patients they need to change their personalities in order to fight their cancer. That is not how it works. How can I be so sure? It's because "I've been there, done that." I've been there and back. Now I recognize that I had a Type C personality at the time of my first marriage. That marriage was a disaster, but I hung in there for 18 years until my health collapsed. I was weak, dizzy, and confused with aching flu-like symptoms that were worse than the flu. I vomited no matter what I ate. Later, I also had uterine cancer, which had developed over the years. I recovered, but it was not because I had a therapist help me change my personality!

Fortunately, as I explain later in this book, I was tested for food allergies and found to be reacting to milk, eggs, wheat, corn, and many other foods. My doctor, following the precepts of Theron Randolph, M.D., had me stay off my worst allergens, use a rotation diet, and lessen the chemical load. By staying off the foods I was reacting to, working on my digestion, and doing all kinds of health building activities, my health gradually improved, and spark came back to my personality.

Dr. Randolph's major book, *An Alternative Approach to Allergies,* was published in 1980 while I was still seriously ill. That book became my lifeline to a better day. Dr. Randolph explained that in the early stages of environmental illness, the immune system causes physical symptoms, but as the immune system becomes more and more disturbed, the symptoms become mental rather than physical. At level III withdrawal, a person usually appears to be just fine. They are slim, active, flexible, and enjoy exercise, but they are often unaware of mental symptoms they may have. Among these symptoms are mild depression, brain fog, impaired memory, indecisiveness, apathy, and difficulty expressing themselves.[101]

When I read Dr. Temoshok's description of the Type C personality, I suddenly recognized myself. That was the way I had been during my marriage. My food allergies didn't suddenly appear when my health fell apart. No, I undoubtedly had them since childhood, especially allergies to milk and wheat. As a young adult, I was already experiencing the mild depression of level III withdrawal. In an unhappy marriage, I was unable to stand up for myself, and I became more and more passive. An unassertive, Type C personality is a symptom of a disturbed immune system that is reacting to all kinds of foods and chemicals in the environment. Personality *does not* depress the immune system.

Dr. Temoshok deserves our gratitude for her insightful research. She has identified a personality type that we can recognize now that she has called our attention to it. The niceness, the desire to appease, the lack of anger, the excessive worry about others, and the guilt all ring true. I used to wonder why I wasn't angry. I would even pat myself on the back for not harboring resentments, but the anger, in reality, just wasn't there. I would add one other personality trait, a poor memory, to the cluster of Type C characteristics. The Type C personality is one type among many under the larger umbrella of level III withdrawal.

About 75% of the melanoma patients Dr. Temoshok interviewed had a Type C personality. One in four Americans die of cancer. One in three has cancer in their lifetime. That means there are millions of people with a Type C personality. This may be the root cause of political correctness.

THE HEALTHY PERSONALITY

LET'S ILLUSTRATE THE LIFE PATTERN OF ALLERGY Man from the outstanding teenager to the heavy middle-aged man to the frail elderly man with a prolonged degenerative disease. Now we will add the life pattern of a healthy man who is not overstimulated by foods and chemical reactions. I will call him Ralph, and Allergy Man will have the name Paul. Even as a baby, Paul is in a hurry. He is strong. He grabs the furniture to propel himself forward, and he skips crawling.[102] Ralph, the healthy man, takes longer to develop. He goes through the crawling stage and takes longer to walk than Paul. Ralph tends to be calm and respectful to his parents as a child, while Paul seems rather hyper, bright, and strong-willed.

During the teenage years, Paul, the Allergy Man, really shines. He is friendly, outgoing, and energetic. He loves the limelight. Paul's energy and aggressiveness give him an advantage in sports. Ralph is a good student, but he is content to watch from the sidelines. He doesn't feel any need to push himself forward. Ralph finds that he has an edge in sports that require endurance such as long distance running.

It is in young adulthood that Ralph begins to come into his own. He is competent, dependable, and hardworking. In fact, he is just the kind of young man employers are seeking. At stimulus level II, Paul is beginning to have problems. He is gaining weight and becoming more aggressive. At this level, some people have the energy, drive, common sense, and charisma to become great leaders. Think of Winston Churchill during WWII. People at this level are natural leaders. Many of the mayors, school board members, and businessmen across our nation fit this pattern. However, another example of a person at level II stimulus might be a used car salesman. Paul has to be practical. He decides to accept a job as a salesman.

We can learn about Ralph and Paul in mid-life in greater detail because Drs. Friedman and Rosenman wrote about them 35 years ago in *Type A Behavior and Your Heart*. They described actual acquaintances of theirs only changing a few details to protect privacy. Paul, who corresponds to our Allergy Man, typified the Type A personality of an overstimulated personality, and Ralph had a healthy personality, which they termed a Type B personality. These two doctors recognized that Paul was overstressed in some ways, was more likely to have a heart attack, and was not as healthy as Ralph was.[103]

Paul Crimmins is the successful manager of a California brewery. He was first hired at the brewery as a salesman 25 years ago. Paul is 52 years old, of medium

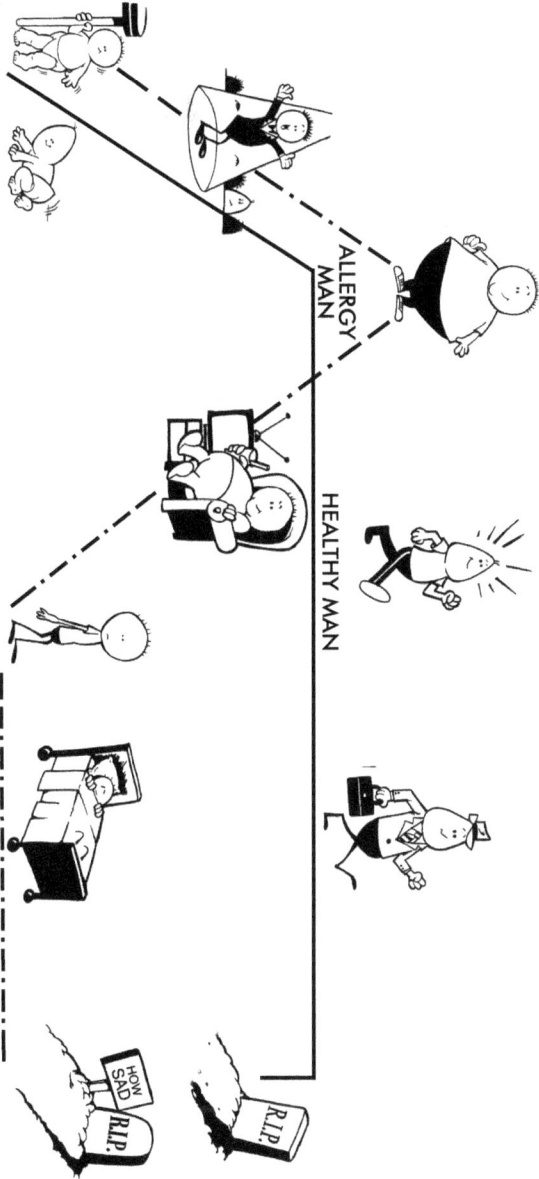

LIFE PATTERNS

A PARTIAL ILLUSTRATION OF THE RANDOLPH PARADIGM

(Modified by the author, MaryAlice E. Bonwell)
DECODING THE ENIGMA

ALLERGY MAN

HEALTHY MAN

© BONWELL   Drawings by Jim Mathenia

height, and 25 pounds overweight. He is married with two adult sons in college. Paul never has enough time. He is always hurrying to get more done. "How can I move faster and do more and more things in less and less time?" is the question that is always with him. He hurries in his thinking and in his speech, and it annoys him if other people get in his way or slow him down. It irritates him if others speak slowly or don't get to the point, and he is angered if the driver ahead of him doesn't go fast enough. He multitasks and does more than one thing at a time as often as he can.

This is before the days of social media, but Paul still has dozens, perhaps hundreds, of friends. These are almost all people he has met in his business life. He strives to have a large network of contacts. However, these are really acquaintances rather than actual friends. He has no problem finding someone to go to lunch or play golf with from his many acquaintances, and he does not perceive a need for close friends.

All of Paul's energies are focused on business. He has almost no hobbies, although he does like to watch football on TV. He just doesn't seem to have time for outside activities. He often brings a trade journal with him to the dinner table. He is easily bored by conversation not about business. He has developed a habit of only half listening when someone, especially his wife and children, are talking about things that don't interest him. He and his wife manage to tolerate each other fairly well, although he finds his wife rather dull.[104]

Ralph Longly is the president of a California bank. He was first hired as a bank teller 34 years earlier. He is 54 years old, rather tall, and weighs the same amount as he did when he played on the baseball team of his university. He is married and has two daughters and one son, all of whom are now married.

Ralph doesn't feel the kind of time pressure that drives Paul. Ralph is a very patient person. It doesn't occur to him that somebody talking with him should speak faster or stop wasting his time. If his flight is delayed, he enjoys reading a book or looking at the magazines in the gift shop. If he has to stand in line, he resigns himself good-naturedly to the wait and observes those around him with interest. He doesn't feel a need to multitask, and he focuses on one task at a time. Unlike Paul, who doesn't think he has time for exercise, Ralph does calisthenics every day. He tries to walk at least 40 minutes a day, and he plays several sets of tennis doubles twice a week with three friends near his own age.

Ralph has five close friends. He goes out of his way to build and maintain his relationships with these friends. He would not hesitate to ask a favor of one of these friends because he in turn would not hesitate to do one of them a favor. Ralph is always courteous and gracious to the men he meets through his profession, but he doesn't attempt to include them in his social life unless he has a particular affinity for one of them.

Work does not consume all of Ralph's time. He has several outside activities. He uses an antique hand press to print books. He has also collected a variety of reference books that allow him to find at least a little information about almost any subject. He enjoys listening to classical music. Both Ralph and his wife take an active interest in live theater. They will drive a considerable distance to see a favorite play performed. Ralph has tried hard to be a good husband and father. He and his wife are still close. They share little things that happened during the day each evening when Ralph gets home from the bank.[105]

To look into the futures of these two men, let's return to our illustration of the life patterns of Paul, the Allergy Man, and Ralph, the Healthy Man. So far, Paul has been on the stimulus side of his allergies, but he will soon lose the energy that has been so much a part of his success as a businessman, and he will go down the withdrawal side of his reactions. At level II withdrawal Paul will probably become a couch potato because of allergic fatigue. According to Dr. Randolph, allergic fatigue seems to be without cause and is not relieved by rest. "It is basically quite unpleasant."[106] Paul will have a hard time hanging on at work until he reaches retirement. Not long after he retires, Paul is likely to begin losing weight at level III withdrawal. In his late 70s, he may begin showing early signs of a degenerative disease such as Alzheimer's disease or Parkinson's disease.

Ralph doesn't go through the ups and downs of life that beset Paul. Virtually all his adult life, Ralph has been on an even keel, the same competent, dependable, resilient person. When I think of a healthy personality, I think of my brother David. The best word to describe him is *steady*: steady weight, steady energy level, steady emotionally, steady intellectual capacity. He has always been someone you could count on. Like Ralph, all of his life he has been the same weight that he was when he graduated from the university. He does calisthenics every day and jogs several times a week.

David is a Christian. He usually doesn't say much about it, but if challenged, he will defend his faith or share it if the opportunity arises. He has always had a few close friends rather than many acquaintances. With him, a close friend is always his friend. He has maintained his friendships with three friends from high school and university days all these years despite living on the other side of the country. He has always had the energy to stay organized, be productive at work, and keep up with his wife and three sons. His family has always come first. He and his wife still enjoy ballroom dancing. You know he wouldn't be angry just because you missed your plane for some dumb reason or because some driver was going too slowly. He did not burn out halfway through his career as a physicist. He is involved in his research and not anxious to retire. Each year I ask him when he is going to retire, and he says, "Maybe next year." Next year will be his 70th birthday, so maybe that will be the year.

How can we tell who has a problem with allergies and food intolerance and who doesn't? Is it simply that a fat person has the problem and a thin one doesn't? No, there are two stages of the Randolph paradigm when a person is thin, at both level I and level III. In our illustration, we see the talented, slim, charismatic teenager at level I stimulus and our poor, thin, little guy at level III withdrawal. Level III stimulus, which is not illustrated, is also a thin stage. A thin person could be healthy, or at the level I celebrity stage, or at the thin level III stage.

It used to be, especially in the WWII generation, people who were reacting to foods and chemicals spent most of their lives on the stimulus side. They were outstanding as teens and young adults. Then, during middle age, they gained a moderate amount of weight. It wasn't until retirement that they hit level III withdrawal and began to lose weight. By that time, losing weight seemed like a natural part of aging.

As we have declined, each generation has had more people who reach level III withdrawal at an early age. What are they like? Remember, at this level people are affected mentally more than physically. They are thin, energetic, and enjoy running, yoga, and other exercise so they seem to be the picture of health. However, they may suffer from anxiety, depression, guilt, poor memory, and feelings of helplessness. Jean Twenge, the author of an important study on American anxiety from 1952 to 1993, found that "the average college student in the 1990s was more anxious than 85 percent of the college students in the 1950s."[107]

In earlier chapters, we have discussed examples of level III withdrawal thinking, such as a diminished sense of humor, an affinity for animals, and the tendency to fasten onto a cause and carry it to extremes. We know that millions of people are at level III withdrawal because depression, vegetarianism, anorexia, and a Type C personality all occur at this stage. These conditions are each discussed elsewhere in this book. As mentioned, many more women than men are at level III withdrawal.

Those at level III stimulus gain an advantage from their environmental reactions. There are more men than women on the stimulus side. These people tend to be slim, smart, aggressive, energetic, self-centered, narcissistic, and controlling. They should not be confused with a truly healthy personality. Their mental capacity is enhanced, especially in the areas of speed, memory, and visualization skills. There is actually a measurable increase in ability. IQ scores in the United States increased by an average of three points per decade during the 20th century. IQs themselves have not risen since each new version of a test is recalibrated so the average score is 100. However, if an unadjusted scale were used, the increase would be substantial.[108] The increase in IQ scores is known as the "Flynn effect," named after James Flynn, a political scientist in New Zealand who discovered this phenomenon in the 1980s. He found test scores were increasing in virtually all the developed world. He worked with data from 20 countries, which includes the United States, Canada, Israel, Japan, and many European countries.[109]

Flynn argues that, compared to our parent's generation, the number of people who score high enough to be considered as "genius" has increased more than 20 times. This means we should now be seeing, as Flynn put it, "a cultural renaissance too great to be overlooked." While we have seen great advancement in technology, it hardly feels like a "renaissance" with the cultural decay we see around us. Flynn suggests that what has risen is not "intelligence" but some kind of "abstract problem solving ability." What I would frequently see with my special education students was an above average score on the performance (non-verbal) part of the IQ test with a below average score on the verbal part. With an autistic child, we might see a spike in one subtest, such as visual memory, combined with low verbal scores. It is the verbal score that correlates most closely with academic success. The increase in IQ scores is most apparent in tests measuring the ability to recognize abstract, non-verbal patterns. Tests based on traditional academic knowledge show much less progress.[110]

What has caused the Flynn effect? The answer usually given is improved nutrition over the last 150 years. Considering that the Standard American Diet is often referred to as SAD, this hardly seems persuasive. Later, we discuss the ways in which the health of virtually every group that has transitioned from natural, traditional food to the diet of Western civilization has degenerated. Poor nutrition rather than good nutrition may be causing some areas of our brains to be overstimulated. Self-described geeks are one group found at level III stimulus. Geeks are known for their love of candy, caffeine, and fast food. At one of the leading hedge funds, the management provides a room full of racks of every kind of candy. All of this is free for the firm's genius mathematicians who are around at all hours and need a sugar high to keep going.[111] Those looking for the cause of the increase in certain mental abilities need to consider the stimulus side of the Randolph paradigm.

The increase in certain non-verbal abilities may be coming at the expense of the emotional and spiritual parts of our personality. To see where this trend may be taking us, consider a young geek in high school. He is thin and smart, two of the most admired attributes in our culture, but he is socially awkward. He misses social cues and doesn't know how to respond to the other kids. If we carry these trends to extremes, we come to autism at level IV stimulus. Here, emotions are limited, and the emotional connection to others is broken. Now let's look at a successful middle-aged man at the beginning of level III stimulus. He sometimes thinks of himself as Mr. Spock of *Star Trek* fame because he prides himself on his rationality. He avoids the emotional side of life. As this stage progresses, people often become increasingly narcissistic and lack empathy for others. He or she may become demanding and controlling to the point that his or her spouse and children become afraid. This is most likely to happen if the overstimulated person is reacting to chemicals.

The heightened abilities of some on the stimulus side may also come at the expense of their spiritual nature. Anthropologists have never found a community that did not have a religion, but we now have many very smart people who seem to have lost their souls. They do not believe in God and are antagonistic to all religion, especially Christianity. There is an old hymn that contains the line "in your heart you know it's true." It is that sense of a connection to God that is being lost.

It's not easy to identify someone with a healthy personality who is not reacting to foods and chemicals. Most of us are very good at faking "normal." Look for someone with commonsense and patience and avoid those who are easily irritated and narcissistic. Having a few close friends and a loving family is an important clue. The healthy person should have a variety of interests and not be easily bored. This person should not be too thin or too fat but just right. As I described Ralph earlier, a healthy person is the one who is on an even keel and is competent, dependable, and resilient.

CLEO: THE STOMACH AND HEALTHY AGING

WHEN I RETIRED FROM TEACHING IN California, I decided to return to my roots in the Pacific Northwest. I was born in Seattle, went to high school in Edmonds, Washington, and I graduated from the University of Washington. Bellingham, or perhaps one of the small towns near Bellingham, seemed like a possible retirement haven. In response to my inquiries to these towns, the Lynden Chamber of Commerce sent a lovely information packet. Lynden is a town of about 10,000 people, which was settled by the Dutch. It is nestled in an area of dairies, raspberry farms, and blueberry farms about 12 miles north of Bellingham, almost on the Canadian border.

During Easter vacation, I flew to Seattle and drove north to Whatcom County to explore the area. As I drove into Lynden, it was a beautiful day. The oak trees lining Front St. were leafing out. The street was lined with charming craftsmen homes with manicured green lawns. It was April, and the tulips were blooming. I passed two beautiful churches and reached the historic center of town with a picturesque Dutch windmill and quaint shops. This was the place for me.

To my delight, I was able to buy a small, but authentic, craftsmen home built in the 1930s. It was only two blocks from the windmill. My first visitor was Margaret, the elderly lady who lived across the street. She came with a plate of cookies. She was warm and friendly. We enjoyed each other. A few days earlier, while I was on the phone arranging for a lawn service, I had observed Margaret mowing her own lawn with a gas powered, push lawnmower. I was surprised to learn she was 83 years old. As I have gotten to know more people, I was impressed with how many robust, healthy seniors were still active in the community.

Lynden is known for its churches. It is sometimes laughingly said there are more churches per capita in Lynden than in any other town in the nation. These are not "museum" churches. The parking lots are full, and they have active congregations. Many of the Dutch belong to a Christian Reformed Church. I found a home in Grace Baptist Fellowship. Almost everyone does more than attend Sunday service. There is Sunday school, Sunday evening service, Bible study, prayer meeting, care groups, and all kinds of social groups. Some of the widows and single older women in the church had formed a fellowship group, which they called Christian Golden Girls. This group met once a month for breakfast at Dutch Mother's restaurant to celebrate birthdays and enjoy each other's company.

The first time I went to Christian Golden Girls, our birthday girl was Cleo Hanlon. Cleo was our oldest member. This was her 94th birthday. There weren't any other September birthdays, so she had the floor to herself. Cleo began telling us about growing up in the little town of Viola, Kansas, near Wichita and her years teaching in a one-room schoolhouse. She had so much personality and was so animated and energetic that I began to wonder what her secret was. Why did she have such a youthful personality?

I happened to be sitting next to Cleo. I looked to see if she had large earlobes. Many elderly women who are still healthy in their 90s have large, plump earlobes, which they hide with big clip earrings. If Cleo had had earlobes like that, I probably wouldn't have looked any further, but her lobes were not particularly good. When she sat down, she placed her hands flat on the table. She had beautiful hands with long slender fingers, nice nails, and not a single age spot. Age spots are usually signs of low stomach acid. Her hair was gray, not white, and unusually thick. In women, thick hair and nice fingernails are important signs of good stomach function. Cleo also had signs of sufficient iodine. Her hairline had not receded, and she had thick eyebrows all the way to the tips. A common sign of inadequate iodine is eyebrows that are thick toward the center but sparse at the ends. Dry hair and skin are also often signs of an iodine deficiency.

Jonathan Wright, M.D. has found that women with a lack of hydrochloric acid in their stomach have either thin hair or weak fingernails. They usually have one problem or the other, but not both.[112] A few months later, I told Cleo's daughter I would like to take some pictures of her mother, especially of her hands, and that I wondered about a manicure. She said her mother had always had beautiful fingernails and would not need a manicure.

As I was looking at Cleo, I suddenly realized that she had deep wrinkles. I said to myself, "That's it. That is the reason." My mind went back to an incident that had happened when I was caring for my mother who had Alzheimer's disease. We were riding slowly around town when an elderly neighbor stopped us and came over to our car. Alice was sharp as a tack, but her face was very wrinkled. She complimented Mother on her beautiful complexion. She went on and on about how beautiful Mother's skin was. Of course, Mother didn't know who this woman was, but she was very good at "faking it." It was true. Mother did have a lovely complexion with almost no cheek wrinkles. As Alice went on about how envious she was, I sat there wondering why Mother had such nice skin when her brain was being eaten away while Alice, who was mentally intact, had many wrinkles.

When I looked at Cleo, it struck me that perhaps the healthy women were the ones with wrinkles. Immuderm, a face cream, which I had purchased, gave me some insight into why this might be true. This face cream was supposed to diminish the appearance of fine lines and wrinkles by stimulating the immune system in the skin. It actually worked. Could it be that smooth wrinkle free cheeks in an older woman indicate an overstimulated immune system and high levels of inflammation? Among women it has become popular to say "fifty-five is the new thirty" because so many middle-aged women look so much younger than they used to. Perhaps this is a mixed blessing. (Wrinkles are not always a good sign. For example, people at level III withdrawal sometimes have many fine facial wrinkles.)

Are thick hair and cheek wrinkles signs of healthy aging in women? I started looking at some of the other women. There were about 20 of us sitting around a long rectangular table. Our ages ranged from 65 to 94, but most were in their 70s and 80s. A few of the women had already been diagnosed with an autoimmune disease or early Alzheimer's disease, and in those ladies, I saw the same smooth cheeks I had seen in Mother. However, most of the women were doing very well and a surprising number did have thick hair and cheek wrinkles. The prevalence of thick hair among these vigorous older women was of particular interest as an indication of the importance of a strong stomach in healthy aging.

At our next monthly meeting, there were 18 ladies present. I let them know how impressed I was by their good health. I asked them how many of them had lived on a farm. Nine had lived on a farm as a child. Then I asked how many had parents who had lived on the farm. All but three had parents who had lived on the farm. I was one of the three. They spoke about drinking raw milk and eating grass-fed beef because that is just the way it was.

The older generation in Lynden came from parents who were still eating natural, traditional foods. Much of this food they had raised themselves. Most of the people in our big cities are at least two or three generations further from the farm. When I first moved to Lynden, I was almost shocked to see how healthy the older people were compared to the people I had known in Southern California. These people do not have the "hurry sickness." They can take the time to answer a question, stop for a pedestrian to cross the street, or wait for a car to move out of its parking place. You know that if you fell on your morning walk, someone would stop and help you. There is still a sense of community and connectedness, but this is disappearing in many places in the United States.

Cleo lived with her daughter and son-in-law. They had turned their master bedroom into an attractive suite for Cleo. However, Cleo was somewhat isolated from the family, and there were long stretches when she was by herself. I was impressed with her attention span and her ability to entertain herself. She liked to watch basketball games. The players she and her husband had watched together were long gone, but she liked to follow the coach. She was interested in people and sent money every month for a little girl in India.

I used to take Cleo for rides because I remembered how much my mother had enjoyed riding in the car. Cleo was more interested in having someone to talk to than the ride. One day we got onto favorite foods. Cleo said she had always eaten a lot of cabbage. In her parent's home, they had made sauerkraut. They usually cooked it and packed it into quart jars. Her mother was Dutch, and her father was Welch, but later, when she taught school, she had been in a predominantly German area. The German families used bigger crocks. Most of her children in school ate sauerkraut. She had eaten sauerkraut all her life. She had also eaten lots of coleslaw and boiled cabbage. She always had coleslaw for company. I asked her what she liked to order in a restaurant. She said she usually ordered a big roast beef sandwich. She would cut it in half and take half home so she could have two big meat meals. She wanted me to know she didn't cut the fat off everything either! Cleo mentioned one other thing that had contributed to her longevity, but this had to do with exercise rather than food. She had been into ceramics. She had her own kiln. She said handling the clay and rolling it out had been great exercise.

I started noticing other older women who had the same signs of good health as Cleo. On my morning walks, I would sometimes see Agnes caring for her roses. We would stop and talk. Agnes had lovely thick hair and cheek wrinkles. She also had good earlobes. In oriental medicine, large ears and large earlobes are considered to be positive signs, but a large mouth is thought to be a sign that the digestive system is losing its strength.[113] I mention the mouth because it can be corrected. I used to have a fairly large mouth. People said I had a lovely smile. One day, after working on my diet and taking large amounts of probiotics, I looked in the mirror and saw that my mouth had disappeared. No, not really, but it had gotten much smaller. After all, the mouth is one end of the gastrointestinal track. If the tone of the gastrointestinal track improves, the mouth will be affected. Even more important, probiotics can be used to remove or at least lessen "whistle marks" around the mouth.

The next time Margaret came over, I observed that she had lovely thick, brownish-gray hair and cheek wrinkles. She had brought string beans from her backyard garden. Fortunately, I had a pear tree and a plum tree so I could return the favor with fruit for her to can. One afternoon, I phoned to let her know the plums were ready to pick.

She said she would be right over. I had expected her to send her grandson or maybe her great grandson. When I suggested that we might need help, she said she would bring her sister. Her sister, Wanda, is four years older than Margaret! Margaret must have been about 86 at this time, so Wanda would have been 90. The two ladies appeared, each carrying a rake. They put the prongs of the rakes up into the plum tree and shook hard. The fruit came tumbling down, and we gathered the plums off the ground.

Several years later, I received an invitation to Margaret's 90th birthday celebration. I wasn't going to be home that day, so I asked if I could drop in a few days early. Margaret hadn't changed much over the years. She still had lovely thick, brownish-gray hair and plenty of wrinkles. She was her usual warm, generous self. Her place was neat and tidy without a scrap of clutter anywhere. In response to my questions, she said she was not taking any prescription medicine, and she still drove her car in Lynden but not in Bellingham. I also asked if she still mowed her own lawn. No, she was letting someone else take care of that. Her large vegetable garden had been reduced to the string beans and one tomato plant, but she did take care of the flowers around her house. While we were talking, Wanda came by. The ladies told me about the quilts they were making at church. These were large, practical quilts, which they gave to the Red

Cross, Salvation Army, and the Lighthouse Mission. They thoroughly enjoyed talking with their friends while they worked on the quilts.

As I was leaving, I impulsively asked the ladies if I could see their tongues. The tongue often reveals the health of the stomach. Both ladies had beautiful tongues without even a hint of a crease or a canyon down the middle of the tongue. However, I now had a new problem. After showing me their tongues, Margaret and Wanda thought maybe I should just use their initials rather than their names when I mentioned them. Ultimately, they did decide that it was alright to use their names. These women are modest and unassuming. They don't want to push themselves forward. How different this is from the narcissistic young people of today who will do almost anything to grab attention.

Margaret was becoming an important part of my story. I decided to phone and learn more about her background. Margaret's parents had come from Dutch families in Michigan. They arrived in the Lynden area around 1900. Margaret was one of six children. Her father worked as a mechanic in Lynden, but the family lived on ten acres outside of town. They had cows and other animals, and they raised much of their own food. As a child, Margaret always drank raw milk. Margaret married a young man who also had a Dutch background, Floyd Aasink. Margaret and Floyd had a 60-acre dairy in the Lynden area. The family always drank raw milk. That included Margaret and their four children. Margaret was quick to assure me that the milk was regularly tested. When she was 70, they retired, and she and Floyd moved into town. Margaret was 70 years old before she started drinking store-bought milk!

About four years after moving to Lynden, I got the biggest surprise of my life. Marian, my best friend of 40 years, died quite suddenly of cancer. She and John had been married 49 years. He was devastated. About a year later, he told me that he was going to be in Oregon for a conference and would drive up to see me. (You may suspect what is coming, but I had no idea.) John arrived on the first of October with all kinds of lovely gifts in his car, including a beautiful set of his mother's blue and white Dalton china. It took several days for me to even realize what was happening. Could I give up the safe little life I had built for myself in my charming little house and take a chance on what was being offered to me? What were my true feelings toward John? Then the dam broke and all the love that had been bottled up inside me flowed out to him. There is all the difference between satisfaction and contentment and real love and happiness. We had known each other for years. We knew each other's background, so there was no point in waiting. At the end of our magical October, on October 26th, we got married in my church with a few close friends and relatives. Our marriage has been the happy ending to my story.

THE STOMACH

WE HAVE SEEN THAT THE STOMACH IS IMPORTANT.
Many people have treated the stomach as though it were
just a bag to hold what they swallow. They have cut it,
wrapped bands around it, and taken drugs to suppress its
functions. Now we are learning that a healthy stomach
that produces lots of hydrochloric acid is essential for
healthy aging.

A strong stomach may also provide the key to
controlling allergies and food intolerance. Consider
what causes an immune system reaction. The immune
system reacts to foreign proteins and to things that look
like foreign proteins. Proteins are huge molecules. They
may contain hundreds and even thousands of amino
acids arranged in branches and chains that fold in on
themselves to form compact shapes. Protein molecules
need to be broken apart during digestion so that only
a few amino acids stick together as small peptides.
Peptides of less than eight amino acids in length do
not react with structures involved in the recognition of
antigens, so they are ignored in immunological terms.[114]
These small peptides can easily move through the walls

of the small intestines where the body uses them to build the new proteins it needs.

Suppose the stomach is not functioning well enough to completely digest protein. A large protein molecule containing 20,000 amino acids might slip through, or it might be broken into large fragments rather than small peptides containing four or five amino acids. A food protein can trigger an allergic reaction if it survives the gastric juices unharmed and is absorbed into the blood through the intestine.[115] If the lining of the intestine has been damaged, partially digested protein can escape into the body in what is called the leaky-gut syndrome. What happens to large protein fragments? Do they stress the immune system? Some research suggests that with chronic exposure, such as milk allergy, linear fragments might be important.[116] Could it be that linear fragments also play a part in food intolerance? Food intolerance is most common in foods eaten every day and at least once in three days. A chronic exposure to grains, sugars, eggs, and other commonly eaten food is similar to a chronic milk allergy. More research is needed on the consequences of partially digested protein fragments.

Pepsin is the enzyme that slices apart the amino acids in a protein molecule, but pepsin can't do its job unless the stomach is acidic enough. When food is eaten, hydrochloric acid is secreted by parietal cells in the gastric mucosa lining the stomach. Gastrin also stimulates the parietal cells and promotes HCl secretion. Pepsin is not fully activated unless the stomach acidity is 4 or less on the pH scale. Acids and alkalis are measured by using the pH scale, which ranges from 0 (most acid) to 14 (most alkaline). Water has a pH of 7, which is considered neutral. The HCl secreted in the stomach has a pH of 0.8, which makes it an extremely potent acid. The normal acidity of the stomach between meals is from 1 to 3 on the pH scale. However, the resting stomach pH in people taking acid depressing drugs is from 4 to 7 pH.[117] The breakdown of protein into amino acids by pepsin takes place most efficiently when the pH of the stomach is less than 3. If the stomach becomes less acidic (pH of 5 or higher), no pepsin is activated. For an excellent discussion of how the upper gastro intestinal tract works, read *Why Stomach Acid Is Good For You* by Jonathan Wright, M.D. and Lane Lenard, PhD. The important thing to remember is that pepsin can't break apart protein molecules unless the stomach is acidic enough.

In the first decade of our new century, a team of doctors and scientists led by Eva Untersmayr, M.D. from the Medical University of Vienna has been investigating the digestion of protein in the stomach. It is interesting that this research has come from Austria rather than the United States where the pharmaceutical companies dominate medical research. The Austrian Science Fund has supported this ongoing research.[118] The objective of the first project was to study how the use of antacid medication influences the allergenicity of dietary proteins. Prior to this research, the prevailing medical attitude was that digestible proteins were irrelevant in triggering food allergies. Would the use of antacids make a difference? According to these researchers, that question needed to be thoroughly explored.[119]

To study protein digestion at different levels of acidity, the major fish allergen parvalbumin was subjected to an in vitro digestion pepsin assay. After 30 seconds of treatment at pH 2.0, this fish protein was completely degraded. However, at pH 5.0, the protein was not digested even after 2 hours. Acid depressing drugs elevate the gastric pH to about 5.0. In mice that had been given antacids, there was an increase in numerous immune system markers. The Austrian team concluded that antacids play a part in causing food allergy. The antacids interfere with the digestion of protein by pepsin and prevent protein molecules from being broken apart into small peptides and amino acids. They concluded, "Our data strongly suggests that medication with antacids puts patients at risk of allergy developing against newly introduced food antigens."[120]

In later research, Dr. Untersmayr and her group found that codfish proteins were degraded within one minute in simulated gastric fluid. It only took a marginal change in pH from 2.5 to 2.75 to completely prevent the digestion of cod allergens. The cod proteins that had been completely digested had a 10,000 times reduced allergenic potency.[121] In the case of milk, it only took an increase in pH to 3.0 for the complete inhibition of protein digestion.[122]

In order to study the effect of anti-ulcer drugs on humans, Drs. Untersmayr, M.D. and Jensen-Jarolim, M.D. observed 152 patients with dyspeptic disorders being treated with antacid medication. An increase in antibodies was confirmed by positive skin tests and oral-provocation tests. Twenty-five percent of the patients had an increase in IgE formation to foods in their daily diet. In those patients who already had food allergies, "… the allergenicity of allergens were reduced up to 10,000-fold by gastric digestion."[123]

Many people who have never used antacids have poor stomach acid production due to inflammation caused by food allergies. According to Dr. Jonathan Wright, the question of whether low stomach acid causes food allergies or food allergies cause low stomach acid is a chicken-and-egg problem. There is a vicious cycle in which allergic reactions to food cause inflammation in the stomach and the lining of the intestine. This reduces HCl secretion and promotes allergic reactions all over the body. When the stomach lining gets inflamed, the parietal cells, which produce HCl, die. For example, when children continue to drink milk even though they are allergic to it, the damage to their stomach lining may be enough to cause gastric atrophy.[124] Researchers in Poland have been able to see localized swelling and irritation of the gastric mucosa after they dripped individual foods through a gastroscope into the stomach.[125]

In addition to acid depressing drugs and inflammation caused by allergic reaction, there is another major cause of inadequate stomach acid. The culprit is *Helicobacter pylori*. *H. pylori* are bacteria that have the ability to survive in the highly acidic environment of the stomach. It secretes a cloak of ammonia and bicarbonate, which neutralizes the acid around it and breaks down the normal mucosal lining of the stomach. *H. pylori* are well known as the cause of ulcers. However, when located in the main body of the stomach, the damage to the lining of the stomach is the most destructive. Some people are not aware of any discomfort with an *H. pylori* infection. However, the typical symptoms are a nauseous, boring kind of discomfort. In his book, *Real Cures Healing Series*, Dr. Frank Shallenber O.D. writes that the discomfort is, "Almost like a strong hunger pang gnawing away in the pit of your stomach." Eating some food usually helps, so a person feels driven to eat something even if he goes off his diet. It gets worse if a person doesn't eat anything. This "gnawing sensation" is a sign of inflammation of the stomach lining that can eventually lead to an ulcer.[126]

In her book, *No More Heartburn,* Sherry Rogers, M.D. writes that some people have only mild symptoms from an *H. pylori* infection, but that "in others, the bug can cause insidious, painless rotting away of the stomach lining." According to Dr. Rogers, *H. pylori* can cause the stomach lining, made up of parietal cells, to be dysfunctional (just as eating gluten causes the lining of the small intestines of those with celiac disease to be dysfunctional). In short, it ruins the lining and makes it useless.[127]

As we have already seen, inadequate stomach acid can lead to incomplete protein digestion. This can cause food allergies and food intolerance. However, this is not the only reason that we need a healthy stomach. Sufficient HCl is also required for the utilization of certain B vitamins, especially vitamin B12. The pathway of vitamin B12 from the food we eat to absorption into the body is complex. The parietal cells in the stomach lining are required at two points. Vitamin B12 enters the body bound to animal protein such as meat, eggs, and dairy foods. The parietal cells need to secrete enough acid for pepsin to separate the B12 from the protein. Parietal cells also secrete a substance known as intrinsic factor. In the case of pernicious anemia, the parietal cells are attacked by an autoimmune disorder so that they don't produce intrinsic factor. Intrinsic factor must be attached to B12 in order for the vitamin to be absorbed from the small intestines into the bloodstream.

There now appears to be an epidemic of misdiagnosed vitamin B12 deficiency. More and more people with inadequate stomach function, especially the elderly, are exhibiting mental changes such as irritability, paranoia, depression, and memory loss or neurological symptoms such as frequent falls and clumsiness that stem from a lack of vitamin B12. Doctors often attribute such symptoms to aging or pre-existing conditions such as dementia without checking further. A registered nurse with pernicious anemia has written an outstanding book, *Could It Be B12?* Sally Pacholok, R.N. was first misdiagnosed and later correctly diagnosed with an inherited form of pernicious anemia. Because of her personal history and her nursing background, she became aware that many patients with a potential B12 deficiency were not being adequately diagnosed. She collaborated with Jeffrey Stuart, D.O. to write what is really a wonderful book with the latest scientific information about vitamin B12. The book is full of personal anecdotes, describes many symptoms, and explains the tests that can be used for diagnosis. Information on a highly accurate urine test described in the book can be found at the Norman Clinical Laboratory website at www.b12.com.[128]

Most symptoms of B12 deficiency can be reversed, but they will become permanent if the problem is not discovered soon enough. Some of the personal stories in the book are sad because they involve infants with developmental delays, pregnant women who had babies with birth defects, and elderly patients in nursing homes who were not tested for low vitamin B12 levels until it was too late. Later, we will discuss the role that inadequate B12 may play in Alzheimer's disease.

There is one last consequence of poor stomach function that I want to call to your attention. When B12 is deficient, levels of homocysteine tend to increase.[129] Frequently, both inadequate levels of B vitamins and high homocysteine levels have been preceded by an undetected *H. pylori* infection.[130] Elevated homocysteine is associated with increased risk of heart disease, blood clot formation, a weakened immune system, and other health problems. When a person has a high homocysteine score, he or she is frequently told to eat less meat and eat more leafy green vegetables. However, Michael Eades, M.D., author of *Protein Power*, points out that vegetarians are known for having significantly increased levels of homocysteine and decreased levels of vitamin B12. Vegetarians obviously don't eat meat and eat plenty of leafy green vegetables. Dr. Eades concludes that B12 is the key to a homocysteine problem.[131] We know that a B12 deficiency stems from damaged parietal cells in the lining of the stomach. When I found that elevated homocysteine is associated with a particular medical condition, I thought, "Poor stomach function."

If you suspect that you might need testing for any problems related to your stomach, especially a B12 deficiency, be sure to discuss your concerns with your physician. Here are some additional signs that might alert you to a problem. People lose their taste for meat and other high protein foods. An elderly person will frequently tell you that she no longer eats red meat. Someone with a milk addiction will often rely on dairy products for their protein instead of eating meat. Another clear sign is a canyon-like crack running down the center of the tongue.

Some signs appear to be merely cosmetic, but they actually are warnings of poor stomach function. In the last chapter, we saw the significance of thin hair and soft fingernails in women. Another one of these "cosmetic" signs is dilated capillaries around the nose and cheeks. The next two are worse than cosmetic. These are bad breath (bowel breath) and body odor. When the stomach is not sufficiently acidic, bacteria from the intestine can move into the stomach and colonize. The odor of these bacteria can be detected in the breath.

Other signs of poor stomach function are bloating, belching, and gas immediately after a meal. A person may feel constantly hungry because of poor absorption. Constipation is often a problem. There may also be undigested food in the stool and rectal itching.[132]

Finally, I will end with a symptom that seems to indicate too much acid. There may be lingering heartburn and acid reflux up to four hours after eating. A person usually assumes that he has excess stomach acid and takes antacids. This may be necessary as a temporary measure to protect the esophagus. However, usually acid reflux, commonly referred to as GERD, is another indication of low stomach acid. When the acid is measured, the overwhelming majority of those with acid reflux are found to have too little acid. Dr. Wright has found that even in serious cases, actual testing shows low stomach acid in over 90% of cases.[133] Dr. Shallenberger reports that he has found *H. pylori* bacteria in nearly all of his patients who have reflux disease. Research shows that up to 88% of those with acid reflux have *H. pylori* infections.[134] GERD can be deadly. It can lead to esophageal cancer even in young adults. A person with acid reflux needs to work with his physician to protect the esophagus and determine the cause of his poor digestion. However, he should not be satisfied with a prescription for antacids or something to keep his stomach from producing acid. There will be serious long-term consequences unless the stomach is healed.

The acidity of the stomach can be measured by the Heidelberg capsule test. Each capsule is about the size of a large vitamin capsule, but it contains a tiny radio transmitter and a pH sensor. In his *Nutrition & Healing* newsletter, Dr. Jonathan Wright describes the way the test is conducted at his Tahoma Clinic in Renton,

Washington. The test is done on an empty stomach. The patient swallows the capsule with a little water. The capsule is usually connected to a very thin string, which feels rather like having a hair in your mouth.[135]

Once the capsule reaches the stomach, it measures the acidity of the stomach, and the transmitter sends this information, which is translated into a graphic computer display. Unfortunately, some doctors or technicians stop the test at this point. Dr. Wright explains that it is very important to see how quickly the stomach can recover from a challenge. He uses bicarbonate, which is a natural substance found in everyone's body, to make the stomach alkaline. A normal stomach quickly secretes acid to overcome the alkalinity, and the pH returns to normal. Normal pH is between 1.8 and 2.3. A healthy stomach can overcome a bicarbonate challenge in 20 minutes or less, five times in a row. However, a poorly functioning stomach takes much longer, or in some cases, doesn't return to normal. It takes about 100 minutes or a little longer to complete the bicarbonate challenges. At the end of the test, the patient has the option of letting the capsule pass through the body naturally or pulling it back up. (This may be important in case of a possible obstruction.)[136]

You can get a list of the doctors who perform the Heidelberg test from the company that manufactures the testing equipment: Electro-medical Devices of Atlanta, Georgia (706-745-9698, www.phcapsule.com).

Dr. Wright stresses that it is important for you to make sure that any Heidelberg test you have done includes bicarbonate challenges.[137]

There are several tests for diagnosing an *H. pylori* infection. The urea breath test (UBT) is a safe, easy, and accurate test for the presence of *H. pylori* in the stomach. The patient swallows a capsule containing a minute amount of radioactive urea. If *H. pylori* are in the stomach, the bacteria change the radioactive urea into radioactive carbon dioxide. The presence of radioactive carbon dioxide in the breath means that there is an active infection. After a person has been treated for *H. pylori*, this test can be repeated to be sure there is no longer any infection. There is a modified form of this test performed with urea that is not radioactive.

A recently developed test for *H. Pylori* utilizes a stool sample. Both the breath and the stool sample tests can be used as pretests and posttests to confirm that the bacterium has been eradicated. There is also a blood test that relies on the presence of antibodies. The problem with this test is that blood antibodies can persist for years, so positive results might be obtained from an old infection that is no longer active. It is also difficult to determine if your treatment has been successful.[138]

Note: the following suggestions for improving stomach function are intended for use after a person has discussed his health concerns with his physician and been tested for, or otherwise eliminated, the possibilities of a B12 deficiency, high homocysteine levels, stomach cancer, or other serious health problems that require immediate attention. This is particularly important in the case of an infant or child who has autistic-like symptoms or is failing to thrive. Remember, vitamin B12 deficiency symptoms can often be reversed if they are caught in time, but these symptoms become permanent if too much time has elapsed.

One of the most effective ways to fight *H. pylori* is drinking fresh cabbage juice. One study showed that drinking four cups of freshly squeezed cabbage juice stopped ulcer pain within two to five days. X-rays showed healing of the ulcers within an average of 11 days.[139] Various sources recommend taking anywhere from one cup to one quart of fresh cabbage juice per day. Dr. Shallenberger suggests taking two tablespoons of cabbage juice and one capsule of cayenne pepper on an empty stomach three times a day. This program should be continued for two weeks. He also recommends taking mastic gum at the same time.[140] A very sensitive person may not want to use the cayenne pepper. Many people have been successful with cabbage juice alone. Antibiotics are effective against *H. pylori*. However, *H. pylori* play a complex role in the regulation of leptin, so it is best to keep overgrowth under control rather than eradicating the *H. pylori* completely.[141]

You may want to get your own juicer because cabbage juice needs to be made fresh each day. It is important to get a juicer that is sturdy and easy to clean. I was fortunate enough to "inherit" a Champion juicer. I love it. It is strong, efficient, and easy to clean, but I've never tried anything else. Straight cabbage juice is hard to get down so you may want to juice a little bit of carrot, spinach, celery, or apple together with the cabbage. I've found that drinking cabbage juice helps me get through those diet-killing times of the day such as late afternoon and after dinner. It seems to take away the desire to snack.

There are several important supplements that will improve the function of the stomach. Mastic has been used for thousands of years in the Mediterranean and the Middle East for many digestive disorders from bad breath to ulcers. Mastic gum comes from a shrub that grows on the small Greek island of Chios. When people have tried to grow this shrub in other places with a similar climate, the plants seem to flourish, but they don't produce the same kind of healing resin. Modern research has demonstrated that mastic has antimicrobial properties. It can kill several strains of *H. pylori*, which includes some that are resistant to most antibiotics. In one study, gastric ulcers were healed in five out of six patients within four weeks. Mastic heals the stomach lining, so it can actually reverse the damage done by NSAIDs, such as aspirin, in addition to killing the *H. pylori* bacteria.

There are no significant side effects with mastic.[142] [143] Mastica (Chios Gum Mastic) is available from Allergy Research Group, www.allergyresearchgroup.com.

Licorice root is another plant-based product that has been used to help the stomach since ancient times. However, licorice was known to have side effects such as high blood pressure and heart problems. Modern science has been able to isolate the ingredient glycyrrhizin, which causes the negative side effects. This ingredient can be removed from licorice just like caffeine can be removed from coffee. This product, which became available in the 1980s, is called deglycyrrhizinated licorice or DGL. Do not confuse DGL with licorice candy. The candy may or may not contain real licorice. If it does contain real licorice, the ingredient that causes side effects will still be present.

DGL has the ability to heal the mucus lining of the stomach and the intestines. It can actually stimulate cell growth and help restore normal activity in the stomach. DGL should be taken on an empty stomach because it heals by direct contact with the gastrointestinal lining. Dr. Wright recommends that two DGL tablets should be thoroughly chewed and swallowed with little or no water three or four times daily. The tablets should be taken one hour before or after a meal. DGL can be taken more often if desired.[144] DGL is available from Enzymatic Therapy in both a sweetened and unsweetened form.

Taking mastic and DGL while getting rid of any *H. pylori* infection doesn't seem too difficult. Here is the hard part. At the same time, a person must not eat any foods they are reacting to because these reactions could cause the cells lining the stomach to continue to atrophy. This gets complicated. How are you going to learn what foods you are reacting to? If these are your favorite foods, how will you avoid them? The next chapters on "Testing for Allergies" and "The Diet" will help you understand what is involved. None of this is easy. The things I have been telling you have personally been helpful, but I still discovered that I needed vitamin B12 supplements for a balance problem. Complacency is dangerous. Work with a knowledgeable professional.

Mastic, DGL, and cabbage juice can help heal your stomach, but it will take time before your stomach is producing enough acid to digest protein adequately. Betaine HCl with pepsin, which is available in health food stores, can be used to increase the acidity of your stomach. However, this is where you need to consult a knowledgeable physician. The lining of your stomach could be too fragile to handle additional acid even though the acid is needed. HCl should not be taken by anyone taking certain medications, especially anti-inflammatory medicine such as Prednisone, high blood pressure medicine, and pain relief medication. Any medication use should be discussed with your doctor.

Aspirin, ibuprofen, and other NSAIDs are especially hard on the stomach. These medications, including common over the counter medicine like aspirin, can damage the lining of the stomach. If this lining is damaged, taking HCl could increase the risk of an ulcer or life-threatening gastric bleeding.

The stomach is a vital organ, and a poorly functioning stomach can be improved. It is much better for you to get your information from experienced physicians rather than second hand. If you are seriously thinking about trying to restore the health of your stomach, there are two books you should read. The first is *Why Stomach Acid Is Good for You* by Jonathan Wright, M.D. and Lane Lenard, Ph.D., which I have relied upon heavily in this chapter. The second is *No More Heartburn* by Sherry Rogers, M.D. Dr. Rogers is a longtime friend of those with environmental illness and autoimmune diseases. In fact, she specialized in allergy, immunology, and environmental medicine. She is the author of the *E.I. Syndrome* and other important books.

Those who have been fighting asthma or depression in addition to food and chemical intolerance must read these books. There is hope for these intractable conditions. Dr. Wright explains the asthma connection and tells how to improve a fragile stomach to the point that HCl can be used. Dr. Rogers talks about Candida overgrowth, intestinal dysbiosis, the leaky gut syndrome, and much more. She even explains how to use a common over the counter product to eliminate *H. pylori*. These books are quite different, but they are both important.

On the Weston A. Price website, www.westonaprice. org, Thomas Cowan, M.D. discusses a different type of program for strengthening the stomach. According to him, low-carbohydrate diets "have been used successfully in virtually all stomach disorders." This is a powerful therapy because the production of stomach acid is closely connected to insulin levels. A person should consume less than 40 grams of carbohydrates per day the first week and less than 75 grams per day thereafter. Dr. Cowan also suggests consuming soup broth with extra gelatin at each meal and drinking beet kvass (www.westonaprice.org/ask-the-doctor/gastorparesis). Unflavored gelatin can be purchased in bulk at www. greatlakesgelatin.com. Smaller quantities are available from www.elitealternatives.net.

William J. Rea, M.D., director of the Environmental Health Center in Dallas, Texas, has found that a large proportion of the patients at the Health Center with chemical sensitivity have low stomach acid. Writing in 1992, he said, "Whether this is part of the problem or concomitant is unknown." This question still is not decided. However, the work of Eva Untersmayr, M.D. and her group has helped to explain the role that low stomach acid plays. Dr. Rea has also found that poor gastrointestinal flora and vitamin B12 deficiencies are a problem among the chemically sensitive. Many of these patients have benefited from B12 injections.[145]

Many of us who react to foods and chemicals have learned that our ability to digest foods is not good. The Woodlands Healing Research Center in Quakertown, Pennsylvania has found that, "A poor, weak digestive system seems to accompany nearly all of our environmentally ill patients."[146] The importance of improving the intestinal flora can't be overestimated. The research in this area is exciting. However, adequate acidity in the stomach is essential for the health of the entire digestive tract. I have observed that those with strong, hydrochloric acid producing stomachs seem to be sturdy individuals who don't worry about their immune systems or their good health.

TESTING FOR
FOOD ALLERGIES
(FOOD INTOLERANCE)

SO YOU WANT TO BE TESTED FOR FOOD allergies, or perhaps you want your child tested for allergies? Please remember that we are talking about food intolerance, not food allergies. (Among friends, you can talk about your "allergies.") This distinction goes back to the bitter controversy mentioned earlier in this book between clinical immunologists and clinical ecologists over the meaning of the term *allergy*. Early in the last century, it was decided to narrow the meaning of the term *allergy* to reactions that involved the immune system and could be demonstrated by the skin-prick tests used by the clinical immunologists. The only legitimate subjects for study became hay fever, asthma, constant runny nose, hives, eczema, and the very violent reactions to foods that can include anaphylactic shock because patients with these conditions were likely to give positive skin-prick tests.[147]

Later, when the clinical ecologists used different methods of testing to uncover *delayed* or *masked* food allergies that could cause a myriad of symptoms, these were not accepted as being real *allergies*. According to clinical ecologist Charles McGee, M.D., hidden food allergy does not trigger the standard immunological test responses such as elevation of Immunoglobulin E (IgE), but significant changes are found in other aspects of the immune system including the serum complement system (especially the C-3 and C-5 components), T-lymphocytes, and total eosinophile counts.[148] Clinical ecologists continue to use the term *allergies* in its original, broader sense of *altered reactivity*. However, the medical establishment does not accept this and prefers the term *food intolerance*.

First, you need to find a doctor who believes food intolerance is fairly common and causes many different symptoms. If you go to a doctor who does not believe that food intolerance is real, he is not likely to find that your depression, nausea, or other symptoms could be caused by something you are eating. According to Jonathan Brostoff, M.D., author of *Food Allergies and Food Intolerance*, estimates of the number of people that suffer from food intolerance ranges from 0.3% to 90%. In other words, some doctors think that hardly anyone has food intolerance, and other doctors think that most people have health problems caused by common foods that they eat. Most orthodox doctors and psychiatrists consider the suggestion that foods or chemical exposures cause mental problems such as depression, anxiety, and hyperactivity quite outrageous.[149]

If you tell your doctor that you want to be tested for allergies, he is likely to refer you to an "allergist" who will probably give you a skin-prick test (also called a scratch test or PSTs), which is done in a series on the back or the arm. These tests work well for some types of allergens, particularly inhalants. However, they are not really useful for foods or chemicals.[150] According to a committee of the Board of Allergy and Immunology, skin tests for foods are only 20% accurate and have little clinical correlation.[151] Dr. Brostoff, M. D. writes that the RAST blood tests are "more expensive, and not significantly more accurate than the humble skin test." [152]

Most people who have had standard allergy testing done assume they have been tested for foods, but they really haven't been accurately tested. One of my special education students was a little boy who was excessively shy and had a serious reading disability. I asked his mother what his favorite foods were. She said that he loved eggs. He had them at almost every meal. I suggested that she have him tested for food allergies. Ultimately, he had a series of scratch tests on his back. The testing did not show that he was allergic to eggs. That was the end of any thought of modifying his diet. It was sad. That little boy probably could have been helped if he had been accurately tested and worked with the right doctor.

There are two new methods of testing for food allergies that are much more accurate than the old blood tests. One is a proprietary stool antibody test from Entero Lab (www.enterolab.com). A test kit can be ordered from this website without a physician referral. The other, from Cyrex Labs (www.cyrexlabs.com), is based on testing the saliva. The lab tests from Cyrex can only be obtained through a licensed healthcare provider. Both websites provide helpful information. Nora Gedgaudas, CNS, CNT, a certified nutritional therapist and author of *Primal Body, Primal Mind,* has had good results using these tests. She especially recommends the Cyrex Labs tests for identifying gluten sensitivity. With all these tests, one has to beware of false negatives. Positive test results are almost always dependable, but a person could, in reality, be reacting to a food that tests negative. [153]

Based on my own experience, the gold standard for testing food and chemical intolerance is the provocation/neutralization (P/N) allergy testing done by clinical ecologists who practice environmental medicine. One food at a time is tested. A drop of allergy extract is placed under the outer skin layers of the arm or dropped under the tongue. The skin test site is observed, the pulse is taken, and the patient's appearance, mood, and symptoms are monitored. Sometimes children are asked to draw or write their name. Then single drops of progressively weaker dilutions of the same extract are given until the patient returns to normal. This dose becomes the neutralization dose that can be used to relieve symptoms.[154] This testing is time consuming and expensive. There are less expensive ways to find out what foods you are reacting to. However, if your family and friends think it is all in your head, your child needs special accommodations at school, or you are being forced to work in a "sick building," then you will be very thankful that there are medical doctors who practice environmental medicine.

Many health professionals use applied kinesiology or muscle testing to learn what foods and chemicals people are reacting to. Applied Kinesiology was originated by Dr. John Goodheart in the 1960s. It was Dr. Goodheart's insightful discovery that there is a relationship between the acupuncture meridians and the muscles. The meridians are the major channels that conduct electromagnetic energy throughout the body. If there is an energy imbalance, it will weaken the related muscles. It is the energy in the meridian associated with a particular muscle that is being tested rather than the physical strength of the muscle.[155] Muscle testing is often used to uncover hidden allergies and learn which supplements will be the most beneficial. In addition to the work of Dr. Goodheart, chiropractors and acupuncturists looked to Chinese medicine to develop kinesiology into a very accurate system for balancing the body's energy and restoring health.

To learn more about muscle testing, go to www. allergyescape.com. The brief tutorial on this website will give you a good idea of what is involved. If you would like detailed information on how to actually perform muscle testing, go to the Price-Pottenger Nutrition Foundation website, www.ppnf.org, for a three-hour DVD, *Muscle Testing for Your Health* by David J. Getoff. You and a friend might try testing each other. This could alert you to factors in your environment that are weakening you. Things like the cell phone you carry in your pocket and the laundry detergent you use can be tested in addition to the trail mix you like to munch on. The real test will be whether you feel better when you give up some of the things that seem to weaken you. I have worked with some chiropractors who were incredibly accurate with muscle testing. However, I would not rely on it to test things my body hasn't actually experienced, such as new supplements.

One of the medical professionals that I consulted with was Dr. Stig Erlander, a Ph. D. biochemist educated in Finland. He had me test for allergies by checking how acidic or alkaline my body was. Your body is more acidic when you react to foods and chemicals. In order to do this test, you need litmus paper or pH paper available from a drug store or online. When urinating, pass the pH paper through the urine stream. If you are acidic, the paper will turn yellowish. If you are alkaline, it will turn bluish.

Use the color code on the container. The problem with this test is that it measures the total load of reactions on the body. You don't know if you are acidic because of the mattress you slept on last night or because of the cereal you had for breakfast. This test works best in a chemically safer, controlled environment.

Probably the most convincing type of allergy testing is the elimination diet. Suppose that one of your favorite foods is oranges, and you want to find out if you are reacting to them. You would eliminate oranges and other types of citrus from your diet for four to seven days. At that time, your body would be very sensitive to oranges if it were a problem food. If you had an orange right at that time, you would have an obvious reaction. In fact, it could make you feel quite sick. This is the form of allergy testing that Herbert Rinkel accidentally discovered when he stopped eating eggs. Five days later, he ate some birthday cake that contained eggs. Ten minutes later, he collapsed on the floor. It took several minutes for him to regain consciousness. Of course, this type of extreme reaction is rare, but it is possible. I would not use this testing with someone who has asthma, heart symptoms, an autistic child who might have a seizure, or anyone with serious or life threatening symptoms.

Dr. Rapp, M.D. cautions that you should never let anyone eat any food if you already know that it causes a severe allergic reaction. Elimination diets are intended to help determine whether frequently eaten foods are causing problems. Only those food items that are routinely eaten should be tested.[156] Let's say that you are obviously better when you go off of milk products for four days. There is no real need to make yourself sick by drinking milk on the fifth day. Continue to stay off of milk for a couple of months and then try having some. At that point, your reaction will be much less. You may not even be aware of a reaction. Don't let that fool you. If you continue to have milk products, your addiction will probably be right back. Always discuss with your doctor which tests would be the safest and most appropriate for allergies and food intolerance in your situation.

As mentioned, the most helpful books on uncovering hidden food intolerance are *Is This Your Child?* and *Is This Your Child's World* by Doris Rapp, M.D. She is board certified in environmental medicine, pediatrics, and allergies. Dr. Rapp realized that provocation/neutralization testing is too expensive and time consuming for many people, so she has always been open to practical, inexpensive ways of uncovering and working with allergies. As she says in the preface to *Is This Your Child's World?*, "This book contains absolutely everything I can think of that might help you to recognize what is interfering with your child's or your own well-being and then eliminate it." Since both these books were written for parents, most adults would not think to turn to these resources for themselves. However, when Dr. Rapp explains how to help a child who is angry or depressed, it is not hard to understand how an adult could be helped in a similar way. When she describes collecting the air in a classroom or in the school lavatory to make an allergy extract it is easy to translate that into air in the workplace or the executive washroom. These books contain typical symptoms of environmental illness, detailed instructions on conducting elimination diets, and helpful methods of recording observations.

What foods are you the most likely to react to? Your favorite foods! That is the sad truth. It is the food that has that perfect, special, just right taste. It's mouth-watering good. Your body actually has the ability to make something you are reacting to taste especially good. It is the food you can't do without. You are addicted to that thing, and your body knows how to get what it wants. One afternoon when I was new to this game, I went for a walk in the park. I stopped at a souvenir stand to find a snack. A small bag of roasted cashews seemed like the safest thing. With the first bite, I knew that the cashews were rancid. The second bite wasn't too bad. By the third mouthful, those cashews tasted great. Later, I found that cashews were a really bad food for me.

An elderly friend of Mother's came to visit us in Jacumba. We told her all about our allergy problems. Helen assured me that she didn't have any allergies. She and I walked to the small, mom and pop grocery store in town to get a few things. As we walked home, she started eating a granola bar that she had just bought. She was disappointed. She told me that the bar was stale. At the end of the next block, Helen turned to me and said that she would have to apologize to our little store. The bar was actually very good. This let me know that she did indeed have some of the same allergy problems that Mother and I had.

The food that you are reacting to the most is the food that you can't do without. When we were planning the reading boxes, I had a business lunch at the Black Angus in Chula Vista with the young man who was going to weld the boxes. When he came in, I noticed that he walked with a pronounced limp. When our food came, he covered everything with black pepper. I suggested that he might not limp if he stopped using pepper. He told me that he would rather die than give up pepper.

What foods do most people react to? Look around the supermarket. The free market economy is really good at giving us what we want, and we really want what we are addicted to. Some parts of the market have changed very little in the last 60 years. Broccoli, celery, and onions seem to have about the same shelf space that I remember as a child. The meat department doesn't seem much bigger. The growth has all taken place in the middle of the store in the aisles of processed food. The manufactured foods made out of wheat, corn, sugar, dairy, processed fats, and artificial chemicals have taken over. The breakfast cereals, potato chips, tortilla chips, candy, ice cream, bakery goods, and sodas have won. Most people with food intolerance find that it is the grain, dairy, sugars, fried foods, and artificial chemicals that they react to the most. The hardest part is that once a person starts reacting to these foods, even pure sugar, pure grain, and pure milk bring on reactions.

The battle for shelf space is very revealing. Usually the most addictive product wins. For years, peanuts have dominated the nut section. Once you get started, it is hard to stop eating peanuts, but have you noticed that cashews have been gaining on peanuts? In some stores, there are now more cashews than peanuts in the canned nut area. Cashews and pistachios are in the same botanical family as poison oak and poison ivy. Could there be something about that plant family that causes us to react to it?

Another battle for shelf space took place between water in glass bottles and water in soft plastic bottles. Soft plastic bottles won hands down. People who had always hated to drink water are now carrying water bottles with them everywhere. The plastic bottle seems to be attached to their lower lip as some people repeatedly sip water. The boring, spring water in #2 plastic, gallon jugs is not keeping up with the soft plastic bottles. Boring is good when it comes to addictions. If you question whether you are reacting to the water in soft plastic bottles, try putting some good (non-chlorinated) water in a handy glass bottle. Notice how often you drink from the glass bottle compared to the soft plastic bottle. Better yet, do not drink any water from a soft plastic bottle for four days and then drink your favorite brand of bottled water. Note: do not forget the cautions given under elimination diets above.

We still want the foods we are addicted to even though we are so full that we can't eat another bite. That is why we are tempted to eat ice cream right out of the carton or have a generous piece of chocolate cream pie after a big meal. Maybe you still aren't quite satisfied after you get home from a big restaurant meal until after you have had a few crackers, some potato chip, or a glass of milk. It is surprising what some people will eat after Thanksgiving dinner. If your daughter-in-law goes to the refrigerator after this feast and gets an orange soda for herself and the children, you know that she is addicted to orange soda. If your daughter-in-law wanders away from the family group after Thanksgiving dinner and goes to the computer, you can suspect that she is addicted to the computer.

Symptoms of food intolerance change as we age. Dr. Rapp shows us the way that symptoms of dairy intolerance change from fetuses, to infants, to toddlers, to children, to adolescents, and adults. For example, in infants that are sensitive to breast milk or milk formula, it tends to cause intestinal discomfort, constipation or perhaps diarrhea, extreme unhappiness with screaming and poor sleep, repeated ear infections, excessive drooling, and perspiration. Some walk early and rock their crib so vigorously that it falls apart. By the time the milk-intolerant individual has become an adolescent, his symptoms have changed, but he is still reacting to milk. This makes his family think that he has "outgrown" his allergy problems, but these problems are just showing up in different ways. Dr. Rapp says that adolescents and adults who couldn't tolerate milk as children usually either love milk or detest milk but love cheese and ice cream. Their main symptoms are diarrhea or constipation, fatigue, irritability, and temper outbursts. They often have hay fever or asthma, which can be caused by dairy as well as inhalants. In time, their milk intolerance can cause them to develop irritable bowel syndrome, colitis, Crohn's disease, tight joints, arthritis, high blood pressure, or heartbeat irregularities.[157]

Symptoms of food intolerance are also different according to the level of stimulus or withdrawal a person is in. My reaction to pomegranates changed as my health improved. When I was teaching in California's Imperial Valley, I had a 50-mile commute from Jacumba. On the way home, I would frequently eat a pomegranate as I was driving. Imagine breaking apart a pomegranate and eating those little red, juicy seeds while you are driving!

I used to tell myself that I must be reacting to them because no one would go through that much trouble unless they were addicted, but I kept doing it anyway. By the time I got home, I had to lie down and sleep for an hour before fixing dinner. Dr. Randolph mentions sleep as a level III withdrawal reaction.[158]

A few years later, after I had retired, I decided to try pomegranates again. I was under much less stress and was doing well on my health program. There was exciting new research on the health benefits of pomegranates. Besides, it is a low calorie treat. Every evening I would eat a beautiful, big pomegranate while watching TV. After several weeks, I started getting pains in my feet. Then the pains got really bad. I could hardly step on my right foot to get out of bed in the morning. It was plantar fasciitis. I knew what it was because there was currently a radio commercial explaining that "first step pain." Sadly, I suspected the pomegranates. As soon as I stopped eating them, the pain vanished. My health had improved to the point that I was getting a level II withdrawal reaction rather than the sleep reactions that I had experienced years earlier. Level II reactions are frequently painful syndromes such as headaches, backaches, nerve pain, and muscle pain.[159]

Look for a pattern of addiction similar to that of a cigarette smoker. The smoker gets a lift from his cigarette, but after a few hours, he craves another one.

Look at the typical person who craves milk. He has milk on his cereal for breakfast and about four hours later has a glass of milk with lunch. In the late afternoon, he has some gourmet cheese with crackers and after dinner enjoys a large bowl of ice cream. Our milk person hardly ever goes longer than four hours without some form of milk. He has learned he will sleep better if he drinks milk before he goes to bed, so at ten o'clock he has a large glass of milk. At two in the morning, he wakes up. He is wide-awake. He cannot get back to sleep. His body is asking "where is the milk?" If he gets up and has some milk, cheese, or ice cream, he will usually be able to go back to bed and go right to sleep.

One clinical ecologist wrote about a patient who craved cantaloupe. This woman would wake up every night at two in the morning. She would be dizzy and have a headache. She could not go back to sleep. If she ate a slice of cantaloupe, all of her symptoms would be relieved. No other food would take care of her symptoms. This woman always had cantaloupe in her house and knew where to buy it during different seasons.[160] My point is not so much to provide a solution to a maddening sleep problem as it is to demonstrate that when you identify a food you crave, you have identified a food you are reacting to. You may be able to eat this food occasionally, but it should be eliminated from everyday use. Otherwise, it will cause long term inflammation and health problems.

Food and chemical intolerance is often behind common sleep problems. It is worthwhile to play detective. Chemicals in the bedroom often make it difficult to fall asleep. Anything from the detergent the sheets were washed in to pesticide sprayed around the baseboards to formaldehyde from the closet shelves could be at fault. Read *The Toxic Bedroom* by Walter Bader to learn about the chemicals often found in mattresses. Nightmares can be brought on by food intolerance. I knew a child who drank excessive amounts of milk and was terribly afraid to go to sleep because of his nightmares. Chocolate and other favorite foods can also cause nightmares. During deep sleep, the tissues in your throat can relax enough that they vibrate and cause snoring. A wife might notice that her husband's snoring is worse during the holiday season than it is in January when he is eating fewer desserts. She might notice that it is worse during pollen season. In that case, an air filter might help. Sleep Apnea seemingly occurs when a person is heavy at level II stimulus and withdrawal. There must be reasons why this develops. Look for the clues.

Just as sleep problems can help us uncover hidden food intolerance so can digestive problems. What happens when we stuff ourselves on our favorite foods? Very often, we have indigestion and even acid reflux. We run for the antacids. When we have a reaction to food, the body turns acidic. Remember, pH paper can be used to test for allergies. According to Dr. Rapp, if some type of alkali such as baking soda or Alka-Seltzer Gold is effective, it is likely that some type of food allergy is present.[161] According to Dr. Rea, "heartburn should be considered a food or chemical reaction until proven otherwise." At the Environmental Health Center in Dallas, doctors have seen a loss of sphincter tone and the triggering of reflux by patients exposed to wheat, corn, sugar, coffee, beef, pork, chicken, and other foods and chemicals.[162] Pay close attention to which foods give you indigestion. Do without those foods, and your indigestion will probably disappear, and your body will have a chance to heal.

I have learned the hard way that the method of cooking can cause food reactions. Food cooked at a high temperature is much more likely to cause reactions than food cooked at a low temperature. Potatoes and olive oil were both strong foods for me, so I grated a potato and browned it in the frying pan. With a little salt, that was really good. How disappointing when I started reacting to this treat! The safest ways to cook are boiling, steaming, poaching, cooking in the crock-pot, parchment paper, or a covered baking dish. With these methods, the temperature doesn't rise above that of steam. Put two large hamburger patties in a covered casserole dish. Place the casserole dish in the oven and cook at 350 degrees for about 30 minutes. Are these patties as tasty as the hamburgers you fry in a frying pan? Probably not! You will not have the fried fat to react to. Which would taste better on your salad, sunflower seeds roasted in oil or raw sunflower seeds? Remember, when you are looking for safe foods, boring is good. Chicken can be baked in coconut milk. Meatballs can be simmered in spaghetti sauce. Wild salmon baked on parchment paper is a gourmet treat. You can still cook delicious food.

Sometimes we put ourselves on an elimination diet without realizing it. We eat something almost every day. Then, without thinking about it, we stop eating it for four days. Maybe we go on a diet or don't get to the grocery store. If we eat that food on the fifth day or soon after that, we could have a bad reaction. That happened to me with chocolate. I had thought that chocolate was an okay food because eating it once in a while was not a problem. I started putting a heaping teaspoon of cocoa powder in my daily smoothie. After several weeks, I decided to add berries and leave out the cocoa. On the fifth day, I had chocolate again. Oh, what a mistake! I was so sick to my stomach. I didn't have any Alka-Seltzer Gold, so I took some antacids. They didn't help. Finally, after four hours of misery, I forced myself to vomit. That helped, but I still slept 11 hours that night. In the Ecology Unit, Dr. Randolph would use alkali salts and milk of magnesia to clear offending substances when a patient had a bad reaction. Oxygen was sometimes used for severe reactions. It is good to keep Alka-Seltzer Gold on hand for just this type of situation. Also look for Alka Aid and Trisalts at the health food store. These products should not be used on a regular basis, only for emergencies.[163]

The food we are reacting to is the food we like too well and eat too much. When a food starts tasting really good and you start wafting it down, you know that it is no longer a safe food for you. Food intolerance becomes food addiction. Food addiction is the root cause of the so-called psychological eating disorders of binge eating and bulimia. A person doesn't binge on broccoli or string beans. They binge on comfort food like cereal and milk, pizza, cake, and ice cream. These foods all contain the grain, sugar, and milk that they are reacting to.

Bulimia nervosa is an eating disorder characterized by binge eating followed by inappropriate methods of weight control including vomiting, excessive use of laxatives, enemas, and compulsive exercising. Ninety to 95% of bulimics are women. More and more young teens are getting into bulimia. About 10% of college women practice bulimia. We can understand this disorder better if we divide it into two types. The first type occurs at level II. This is the stage when a person rapidly puts on weight. He craves the foods he is reacting to, and it takes large amounts of food to satisfy those cravings. A young woman doesn't want to gain weight, but her cravings call her to eat the wrong foods. Once she takes the first bite, it is like the alcoholic who takes the first drink. The compulsive urge to eat doesn't stop until she has eaten way too much. She may try severe dieting, but when this becomes too difficult, she may turn to vomiting. Doing this a couple of times would hardly matter, but the cravings never stop. A pattern of bulimia develops. Some people do it several times a day. The average is about 11 times a week.

The bulimia that occurs at level II follows the classic pattern of food intolerance. A person craves the food he is reacting to. He eats the food. It tastes wonderful. He feels great. A few hours later, he feels horrible and is nauseated. He vomits. He feels much better. He feels fine until the cravings start again. At level II, the symptoms are physical. A person feels miserable until he gets that food out of his body. It is that as much as the desire to be thin that brings on the vomiting.

At level III withdrawal, symptoms are mental rather than physical. Remember the pomegranates. They caused sleepiness at level III and muscle pain at level II. The cravings are also different. The cravings are specific and insistent, but it only takes a little bit of food to satisfy them. People at this stage tend to eat little bits of food frequently. The type of bulimia that occurs at level III withdrawal is usually associated with anorexia. A woman who is already dreadfully thin inexplicably keeps vomiting what little food she does eat so that she can get thinner!

Suppose that an anorexic young woman gives in to her cravings and eats a few cookies. A short time afterwards, she is filled with shame, remorse, and anxiety over what she has done. These are mental symptoms brought on by reactions to the food she just ate. She cannot get over these terrible feelings until she vomits. She must get rid of every morsel of the food she has eaten in order to assuage her guilt, so she wretches and wretches. Once she has gotten the offending food out of her body, she can finally feel calm and peaceful. By the time a person reaches this stage, she is probably reacting to many of the foods she eats. The offending foods could be milk, grain, melon, carrots, pepper, cinnamon, or just about any food.

The health consequences of bulimia are severe. Repeated exposure to acidic gastric juices causes erosion of tooth enamel, dental cavities, and sensitivity to hot or cold food. In addition to other serious problems, it can cause stomach ulcers and ruptures of the stomach and esophagus. About 10% of individuals with bulimia will die from starvation, cardiac arrest, other medical complications, or suicide.[164] A person caught in this trap should look at the No Addiction, Sprouted Grain Diet, or the Paleolithic diet discussed in the next chapter.

We are not helpless. Rich or poor, we can discover the hidden food reactions that are destroying our health. In addition to all the methods of allergy testing discussed in this chapter, I recently became aware of a little test that is surprisingly accurate. Beware of anything that is "mouth-watering" good. At that moment when you give yourself permission to eat something, saliva begins flowing into your mouth. This is part of the normal digestive process, but if a person is reacting to a food the flow will be much greater than if the food is not causing a reaction. Dr. Rapp writes that food-sensitive infants and children may suddenly drool excessively, and sometimes the saliva almost pours from their mouth.[165] Start paying attention to this warning sign.

THE DIET

DON'T WE ALREADY KNOW THE DIET THAT WOULD be best for us? Degenerative diseases were virtually unknown in the isolated groups studied by Weston Price. There was almost no cancer or heart disease among those people who did not use white flour or processed foods. In groups such as the Hunzans and the Okinawans, many centenarians were still active and hard working. They were respected for their wisdom. Alzheimer's disease was unknown. Even in America, health records show that the number of heart attacks per 100,000 people was near zero in 1890. Today 44% of all deaths in the United States are caused by heart attacks, and one in every four men will have a heart attack before retirement age.[166] According to the article "Alzheimer's Disease or the Baby Boomer Nightmare," 50% of people over 85 have symptoms of Alzheimer's or other forms of senile dementia.[167]

Many Americans are trying to return to a more natural way of eating, to a diet that reflects the healthy diets of our ancestors. Organic and locally grown, unsprayed produce is available in many small, fresh food markets, food co-ops, and even in some large grocery stores. Many shoppers will go out of their way to get wild salmon, grass fed beef, and whole grain bread. Wouldn't it be wonderful if we could eat the cheese, cream, and grass fed beef from alpine meadows like the Swiss? We could put the cream on big bowls of slow-cooked oatmeal like the Celtic peoples. We could eat wild fish and shellfish like the Samoans and Okinawans. Apricots and other delicious fruits and vegetables could be picked fresh every day from our own gardens like the Hunza's. Perhaps, if we had not lived on a diet of processed foods for more than a generation or two, we might be able to return to this healthy, natural way of eating. Unfortunately, this idea comes about 100 years too late for most of our population.

Remember Pottenger's cats? By the third generation, 95% of the cats had allergies. We are now at least five generations away from a natural diet. As each generation becomes weaker, more and more people suffer from poor digestion, allergies, and food intolerance. If a person is depressed because he is reacting to wheat, it won't help him to eat stone ground, whole wheat bread instead of white bread. If a child becomes angry and aggressive after eating chicken eggs, it won't matter if his mother buys him fertile, brown, organic eggs instead of white, jumbo eggs. Some, who are reacting to pesticides, additives, and chemicals rather than the foods themselves, will do very well on organic foods. Unfortunately, most people with food intolerance and addiction are disappointed to find out that they react just as much to organic foods as they do to the commercial products. The great effort that has gone into making natural and organic foods available does mean that a person on an elimination diet can find wholesome food. However, most people whose health is being undermined by reactions to many basic foods will not find relief from a well-balanced, natural diet. Even though the food is nutritious, these people will still react to it and suffer from degenerative health conditions.

If a balanced, natural diet is not right for someone with hidden food addictions or intolerance then what are the safest foods? Dr. Randolph has ranked the food types from the most addictive to the least addictive. He places alcohol at the top, and he calls alcoholism the pinnacle of the food addiction pyramid. Next come coffee and cola drinks that contain caffeine, followed by chocolate and tea that contain theobromine. Yes, chocolate really is high on the addiction pyramid! No wonder Starbucks is successful with blissfully sinful concoctions of coffee, chocolate, dairy, and an extra shot of caffeine! The cola drinks and chocolate usually contain sugar. Then come the sugars followed by the starches. The safest or least addictive food types are the proteins and fats. Oils and fats are on the very bottom of the pyramid as the food group least likely to cause reactions.[168]

```
                    Alcohol

                    Caffeine
                     Coffee
                  & Cola Drinks

                  Theobromine
                Chocolate & Teas

                    Sugars

                    Starches

                    Proteins

                  Oils & Fats
```

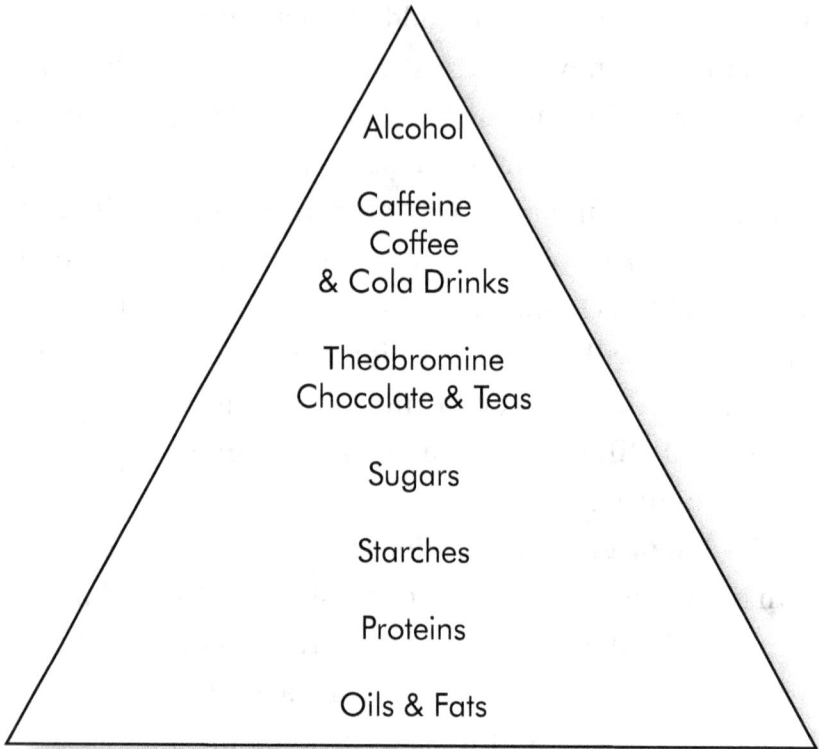

THE FOOD ADDICTION PYRAMID

We crave those foods at the top of the addiction pyramid, especially the sugars and starches. Are you a foodaholic? Too many Americans know what that is all about. We don't feel satisfied until we finish our ice cream after dinner. If we take one cheese cracker, we just have to finish the whole box. If the next meal doesn't come soon enough, we have an all-gone feeling until we grab a snack. That is the way it is at level II stimulus. That is why so many Americans are overweight. The government tells us to eat fewer calories. That means taking less than we want of what we crave. That will never work in the long run.

It is much harder being a foodaholic than it is being an alcoholic. The alcoholic only has to give up alcohol. He can eat food. The foodaholic can't give up food. He has to keep eating, but eating is destroying him. No one would suggest to the alcoholic that he restrict himself to one drink each time he opens a bottle. That one drink would set up his cravings, dissolve his will power, and he would finish the bottle. The low calorie diet demands that the foodaholic restrict himself to eating only a little bit of what he craves. That is like telling the alcoholic to just drink a little bit. Say a dieter is on a 1,200 calorie per day diet. He can have cookies but only 100 calories worth! That is one real cookie or 12 tiny, chemically-laden cookies. Who ever heard of eating only one cookie? But our dieter does manage not to take another cookie. He secretly congratulates himself on not taking a second one. However, three hours later, the craving for wheat that started with the cookie gets too strong, and he goes for a toasted bagel with cream cheese and then another bagel with more cream cheese. Just as the alcoholic must not take that first drink, the food addict must not take the first bite of the foods he craves.

It is easy to pick out the people who are at level II stimulus because they are heavy. We can all understand why a person at this level is dieting. However, another group of people puts themselves on restrictive diets despite already being thin. These people are at level III withdrawal. It is hard to spot a person at level III withdrawal because they appear to be healthy. As Dr. Randolph observed, their symptoms are mental rather than physical. They are thin and flexible and usually enjoy exercise. There are many more women than men at this stage because men tend to go up the stimulus side with their reactions while women go down the withdrawal side. As we have seen earlier in this book, most women at this stage do not like to be looked at. They tend to love animals deeply and will even sacrifice themselves for animals. These women tend to be very sweet, and they cannot bare conflict. However, they will focus like a laser on their cause or goal and will not be dissuaded by reality or common sense.

As we saw in the chapter on a healthy personality, in earlier generations, level III withdrawal came at the end of life. After decades at level I stimulus as a young person and further decades as an energetic, overweight person at level II stimulus, a person became thin and a little anxious and forgetful. This was seen as part of aging, but in reality, these people had entered the stage of level III withdrawal. As people have gotten weaker with each passing generation, an increasing number have reached level III withdrawal earlier in life, even as young adults.

As young as they are, more and more teenagers are already at level III withdrawal. This may be the reason we now have the phenomenon of teenage vegetarians and anorexic young women in the United States and many of the Western, developed countries. According to Mark Penn, author of *Micro Trends*, about 1.5 million children in the United States between the ages of 8 and 18 are vegetarians compared to almost none 50 years ago. Some of these kids are influenced by their vegetarian parents, but more and more are rejecting meat on their own. This is especially true of girls. A surprising 11% of girls aged 13-15 say they don't eat meat. There are now about 11 million vegetarians in the United States. Vegans account for one-third to one-half of these.[169]

Let's look at one type of young girl who is attracted to being a vegetarian. I'll call her Helen. Helen is a slender girl who is pretty, sweet, and sensitive. She loves the beauty of the wilderness and hates to see the world around her taken over by cars, concrete, and ugliness. She loves animals. Helen has poor digestion with low hydrochloric acid (HCL), and also reacts to grain, but she is not aware of either. Because her stomach acid is low, meat does not appeal to her. Her favorite foods are bread, cookies, and macaroni and cheese. Being a vegetarian attracts her. Helen is appalled by the cruelty of killing animals for food. She tends to be a perfectionist and becomes overly anxious about the problems that touch her heart. Giving up meat is no sacrifice. She doesn't like it anyway. Helen will be able to eat as much as she wants of the bread, cereal, and other favorite foods she is addicted to. Besides, her vegetarian friends tell her that a plant diet is much healthier than a meat diet and will keep a person from getting fat. (In reality, vegetarians are thin because they are already at level III withdrawal. A person at level II stimulus would balloon up in weight on a vegetarian, high carbohydrate diet.) There are many young women like this, and they belong to level III withdrawal.

Researchers who have studied young vegetarian women have been puzzled because these women appear to be healthy, but they are more likely to suffer from depression than non-vegetarian women. In 2000, the Australian Longitudinal Study on Women's Health studied 9,113 women aged 22-27. The vegetarian and semi-vegetarian women were thinner and exercised more than the non-vegetarian women. The vegans were the thinnest. The study concluded that although their physical health was good, the mental health scores for the vegetarian women were significantly lower than those of non-vegetarians. Women in the vegetarian group reported more depression and deliberate self-harm incidents. The vegetarian women were also more likely to be taking medication for depression.[170]

A large Scandinavian study of 2,041 teens with a mean age of 15.5 years found that vegetarianism is "mainly a female phenomenon among adolescents." These young women reported having more sick days and were depressed more often than female omnivores.[171]

A study from Finland demonstrates how difficult it is for most people to realize that a person who has depression but appears to be healthy is really sick. Remember that at level III withdrawal, a person loses his or her physical symptoms, but then they start having mental symptoms.

> The results showed that vegetarian and semi-vegetarian women had a lower self-esteem and more symptoms of depression and eating disorders than omnivorous women. In addition, vegetarian women had a more negative view of the world than semi-vegetarian or omnivorous women did. The results suggest that although vegetarians may be healthier, they may be less happy than other individuals.[172]

Psychotherapist Abigail Natenshon has observed the increasing trend of young people adopting a vegetarian lifestyle, and she has a warning for parents. She has specialized in the treatment of eating disorders for over 30 years and is the author of *When Your Child*

Has An Eating Disorder. Someone with a compulsion to lose weight can use vegetarianism as an acceptable cover. Parents should watch for signs that their daughter is preoccupied with a fear of getting fat, especially if she thinks she is fat when she is not. They should notice if she skips meals and seems to play with the food on her plate rather than eating it. Parents should watch for signs of anxiety such as compulsions, perfectionism, over-achieving, and signs of depression such as social withdrawal, irritability, and difficulty concentrating.[173] Between 30% and 50% of the women seeking treatment for anorexia and bulimia are vegetarian.[174]

Lierre Keith, in her powerful book *The Vegetarian Myth*, has exposed the cult-like appeal of the vegetarian life. This is an easy-to-read, beautifully written, deeply personal, warm, honest, serious, eye-opening book. Lierre (rhymes with Pierre) was a vegan for 20 years. She warns that a vegan diet, especially if it is low fat, is not adequate for long-term health maintenance. Her own health was ruined. In addition to exhaustion and depression, she had constant nausea and pain in her spine, later diagnosed as degenerative disc disease. As she writes:

> Understand the pain level I was living in by then: I couldn't sit for more than thirty minutes or stand for more than ten. Every daily task had to be broken down into the smallest activities,

separated by endless stretches of lying down. One extra load of laundry or a long line at the bank and pain would eat my life to the bone. I could spend weeks lying in bed waiting for it to subside.[175]

Why didn't she stop being vegan and get help?

I read survivor narratives of eating disorders, and I recognize way more than I want to. Is it because we inhabit the same brain, the vegans, and the anorexics?[176]

If you are the parent or the grandparent of a young person who is thinking of being a vegetarian, read *Vegetarian Myth*. Have the doctor check for adequate hydrochloric acid secretion and other possible digestive problems. Read the section on anorexia in the last chapter of this book.

If you are wondering why a vegetarian diet is supposed to be superior, you will be interested in learning how those pushing the vegetarian agenda have manipulated some facts and ignored others. *Myths & Truths About Vegetarianism* is a thoughtful, well-documented article available on the Weston A. Price website, www.westonaprice.org.

Both those on a conventional weight-loss diet and the vegetarians have chosen to eat from the top of the addiction pyramid. They go from one meal to the next eating the foods they love. No one wants to give up the foods they crave. It is hard to pry a person free from an addictive diet. A person doesn't realize that many of her health problems, whether physical or mental, come from reactions to her favorite foods.

There is a diet based primarily on the protein and fats at the bottom of the addiction pyramid. The Paleolithic diet has been inspired by the kinds of foods our hunter-gatherer ancestors would have eaten long before farming started. Early man was a skilled hunter and a meat eater. Anthropologists and archeologists have found that these hunter-gatherers were healthier, more robust, had greater bone density, and had a longer life span than people who lived in the agricultural civilizations that came after them.[177] The Paleolithic diet is high in protein and fat but low in carbohydrates. Picture the food that would have been available. The animals or perhaps the fish that were hunted would provide protein and fat. A small amount of carbohydrates would come from gathering berries and other wild plants. In order to survive a person must have proteins and fats, but carbohydrates are not essential for human health.[178]

There have been groups of people who have lived exclusively on protein and fat for long periods of time. In the 1920s, two explorers returned from the arctic. They reported that Eskimos were able to live on nothing but caribou meat all winter long while doing strenuous work. To prove that this ability was not limited to Eskimos, the two explorers, Vilhjalmur Stefansson and Karsten Anderson, volunteered to be studied and monitored by Bellevue Hospital in New York City for one year. During this famous study, the two men ate a meat diet of more than 2,500 calories per day. Their diet was 75% fat. At the end of the year, both men had lost about six pounds. Their cholesterol levels and other blood chemistry values were normal and neither experienced any adverse effects.[179] [180]

The Masai nomads of Kenya live exclusively on milk, blood, and small amounts of meat from their cattle. In 1962, their blood-cholesterol levels were measured. Their cholesterol levels were among the lowest ever measured. When some of the Masai moved into Nairobi and began eating a traditional Western diet, their cholesterol increased considerably.[181]

High protein/low carb diets such as the Atkins diet have largely been touted as quick weight-loss diets. The Paleolithic diet is much more than that. It is a healthy way of living. The husband and wife team of Michael R. Eades, M.D. and Mary Dan Eades, M.D. has had wonderful success using this type of diet to help patients with many intractable health problems as well as weight loss. The key to their success is the effect of a low carbohydrate diet on insulin. A diet high in carbohydrates stimulates insulin production. Excess insulin is behind our epidemic of type II diabetes, high cholesterol, high blood pressure, and obesity. Most of us are aware of the danger of eating too much sugar. Where we have made a mistake is in thinking sugar is bad but complex carbohydrates are good. All carbohydrates are basically sugar. It may take a little longer, but the body breaks down complex carbohydrates chemically and releases the sugar molecules into the blood. It matters little whether you eat a baked potato or have a soft drink; your body will have to deal with a quarter cup of sugar.[182] In fact, if you eat as most nutritionists suggest—a 2,200-calorie diet that is 60% carbohydrate, your body will have to metabolize almost two cups of pure sugar per day.[183]

In their book, *Protein Power*, Drs. Michael R. and Mary Dan Eades tell us about an iceberg used as a metaphor for hyperinsulinemia. At conference meetings, Dr. Ralph DeFronzo, M.D., head of the Diabetes Division of the University of Texas Health Science Center at San Antonio, draws a picture of a huge iceberg with peaks labeled hypertension, heart disease, high cholesterol, diabetes, and obesity sticking out above the water. The great mass of the iceberg deep under the water, the part hidden from view, he labels hyperinsulinemia. While doctors and patients worry about individual diseases, the great dangerous mass remains hidden from view.[184]

Research has also uncovered a connection between hyperinsulinemia and cancer. It appears to enhance tumor cell proliferation in many types of cancer.[185] Nobel Prize winner Dr. Otto Warburg discovered that cancer cells live almost entirely on glucose. They can't convert fat efficiently. By eating a diet that provides adequate fat and very few carbs, a person feeds his healthy cells while starving the cancerous ones.[186]

The Paleolithic diet doesn't just reduce insulin levels. It also gets people off the foods they are most addicted to. This can reduce inflammation. Those with food intolerance find that it is the sugars and starches that bring on most of their symptoms. The Drs. Eades have found that, in addition to the classic insulin resistant diseases, many other health problems clear up on their low carbohydrate diet. For example, they mention skin rashes, acid reflux or heartburn, difficulty sleeping through the night without getting up for a snack, and sleep apnea. These could well be symptoms of food intolerance. When a patient stops eating foods he is reacting to, these symptoms and many others might disappear. The Eades have a knack for making the complex very clear. They explain how a low carbohydrate diet can build health as well as how it can help us lose weight. They discuss ketones, microhormone messengers, and many other aspects of diet and health that go beyond what I have mentioned here. A person with type I diabetes should not use this diet. Read *Protein Power* and *Protein Power Lifeplan* by Michael R. Eades, M.D. and Mary Dan Eades, M.D. It is exciting to find a simple, workable diet that can help us escape the terrible degenerative diseases that are overwhelming us at younger and younger ages.

It took many years before I found the Paleolithic diet. Perhaps sharing my background will give you a feel for what it was like for one person to cope with food intolerance. My health had collapsed in my late thirties. I felt sick all over with nausea, vomiting, exhaustion, brain fog, and helplessness. I was at level III withdrawal complicated by long-term stress and adrenal depletion. I was so fortunate that my best friend, Marian Bonwell, got me to a clinical ecologist. My doctor was Dr. Charles McGee, M.D., author of *How to Survive Modern Technology*. He diagnosed my food intolerance. I was reacting to all the food groups that were tested. I was a so-called "universal reactor." I was put on a rotation diet. On a rotation diet, you don't have any food family more often than once in four days. That is, you might have grain on day one, sweet potato on day two, beans on day three, and white potatoes on day four. The idea is that the rotation will prevent you from overusing your foods and losing more foods. Food sensitive patients can frequently tolerate test positive foods if they are eaten far enough apart, but it wasn't right for me. [187] For example, I would eat eggs and about three hours later begin vomiting. One especially bad episode came on in the parking lot of Cost Plus Imports when I was out shopping with Marian. I was always nauseated. I even tried a 15-day rotation. That means having only one or two foods a day. A rotation diet will only work if you have enough safe foods to rotate, and I didn't have any safe foods.

One of my doctors suggested that I try eating rabbit since I didn't think I had eaten rabbit before. (As a child, we had neighbors who raised rabbits, so perhaps I had been exposed to rabbit.) After my sample meal of rabbit, I was violently ill with projectile vomiting. Twenty-five years later that incident helped me to discover why I had become a universal reactor. While doing research for this book, I found the following information in Volume 1 of *Chemical Sensitivity*, the impressive work by William Rea, M.D. Dr. Rea is considered to be the leading clinical ecologist in the generation following Dr. Randolph.

According to Dr. Rea, bacteria produce pantothenic acid in the human gut by combining B-alanine and pantoic acid. This step can't be completed without the correct bacteria being present. Without the bacteria, B-alanine becomes elevated. A person with food and chemical reactions with this amino acid abnormality may become a "universal reactor." One way to treat this is to reduce B-alanine sources in the diet. These foods are the anserine and carnosine peptide meats: chicken, turkey, duck, rabbit, beef, pork, tuna, and salmon. That is the reason a proper balance of intestinal flora is necessary in both the food sensitive and chemically sensitive individual.[188] Evidently, I had had inadequate intestinal flora as well as inadequate stomach acid when I became so ill. That is probably the reason colon hydrotherapy treatments and taking large amounts of probiotics proved to be very helpful. Some of my worst reactions were to the meats on Dr. Rea's list. In addition to the rabbit incident, there was an especially bad one to turkey. I had always wondered why I could eat most fish, but not tuna and salmon.

My world had fallen apart. I had to stop teaching. I asked for a legal separation from my husband, but my marriage ended in divorce. My parents had retired to an American development in Mexico on the Baja coast. Sadly, my father had died. Mother was alone. She welcomed me with all the love that only a mother can give. Several things came together to help me get a new start. In addition to being in a stress-free, loving situation, the environment was clean with ocean breezes streaming in. Before leaving for Mexico, I had the mercury removed from my teeth and completed a series of colon hydrotherapy treatments that had stopped the constant nausea. I was also consulting with Dr. Stig Erlander who helped me find a few safe foods. My safe foods were cabbage and other vegetables in that food family, some kinds of fish, white potatoes, and olive oil.

As my digestion improved I was able to eat most meats including tuna and salmon., but I was not really excited about eating meat. What I wanted was sugar and starch. None of the sugars would work whether it was beet sugar, agave, rice syrup, maple sugar, honey, or xlitol. I craved cane sugar the most. Sugarcane is a grain. Molasses is made from sugar cane. Just thinking about a molasses cookie makes my mouth water even now. Only stevia was safe. The starch foods seemed to tease me. I would discover a new food such as yucca root or buckwheat and eat it for several weeks. Just when I was really beginning to like it, my arthritis would flare up, and I would know that I should stop eating that food. It sounds funny, but it is scary too. What if you lose all your foods? Just when it did seem like there were hardly any foods left, something good happened. I discovered sprouted grains and beans.

When grains, beans, nuts, and seeds are sprouted, they become more digestible. Sprouting grains neutralizes enzyme inhibitors as well as the phytic acid that keeps certain minerals from being absorbed. Sprouting also inactivates aflatoxins, potent carcinogens found in grains.[189] A quick Google search revealed that there are many benefits to sprouting and that it is frequently helpful to those with food allergies. Apparently, the gluten grains are not safe for those with celiac disease even after they are sprouted, but celiacs could sprout rice, beans, seeds, and nuts.

For several years, I went on what I called the *No Addictions, Sprouted Grain Diet*. This meant not eating anything I was reacting to and not eating any grains or beans unless they had been sprouted. This means just barely sprouted, about an eighth of an inch long, not a leafy green sprout. This proved to be quite workable and kept my food reactions under control. I would sprout wheat berries (hulled wheat available at the health food store) and cook it overnight in a crock-pot. The next morning there would be the most wonderful cooked, plump, golden grains of sprouted wheat waiting for me. Breakfast would be a cup of cooked, sprouted grain with a sliced banana and coconut milk sweetened with stevia. Lunch would usually be beef or chicken vegetable soup. I usually put sprouted beans in the chicken soup. Sometimes it would be a tuna salad. Dinner would be grass-fed beef, bison, organic chicken, or wild salmon cooked in a covered dish in the oven to avoid frying or baking at high heat. There would also be a vegetable, a fresh green salad, and some sprouted grain or sprouted beans to go with the meat.

The Paleolithic diet promised me the two things I was still looking for: weight loss and lower blood pressure. It seems that insulin causes the arteries to thicken and lose their flexibility. It also causes the kidneys to reabsorb sodium rather than excrete it.[190] This leads to hypertension. Low insulin would also help keep the frightening degenerative diseases of civilization at bay. Furthermore, the diet was based on my strong foods, fats, proteins, and low-starch vegetables. I could hardly believe my good fortune. However, in practice, it wasn't so easy. Because of my food intolerance, I wasn't able to eat eggs, cheese, yogurt, whey and other milk products, or any nuts and seeds. This made the diet very restrictive. However, trying to use the Paleolithic diet showed me that I could easily cut back on carbohydrates.

That is where I was going to end this chapter: frustrated with my combination allergy/Paleolithic diet and defeated by my carbohydrate cravings. Then I read *Primal Body, Primal Mind* by Nora Gedgaudas. Her book takes the Paleolithic diet to a new level. She emphasizes the importance of fat. Fat was highly prized by early hunter-gatherers. Fat makes us feel satisfied, and don't we wish we could feel satisfied!

Eating carbohydrates causes the body to produce insulin. Insulin signals the cells to burn glucose rather than fat. It suppresses glucagon, the enzyme that enables the body to burn fat. Body fat can't be used as fuel as long as insulin is present. What happens if we cut back on carbohydrates and eat lots of protein instead? The body will convert the extra protein, beyond what it requires, to sugar and store it as fat. The body, including the brain, is actually designed to use fat for energy.[191]

These facts lead to a diet based on enough quality fat to feel satisfied, a moderate amount of protein, leafy green vegetables, and maybe a few berries. Even without following the diet perfectly, these principles have been very helpful. With this type of diet, I am achieving the goals that first attracted me to the Paleolithic diet. Nora Gedgaudas is on to something! Before trying this diet, it is important to read *Primal Body, Primal Mind* to understand possible pitfalls and precautions. In this outstanding book, Nora Gedgaudas brings her common sense and her technical expertise to many health problems that are troubling all of us.

There are many advantages to going on a low carbohydrate diet, even if it is only for a short time. Going on the Paleolithic diet for a month or two would be one way to discover if reactions to carbohydrates are undermining your health. Most people will be surprised how much better they feel and look on a diet based on fats and proteins rather than one based on carbohydrates.

MOTHER

I FIRST NOTICED THAT MOTHER WAS BEGINNING to slip when she came to visit me in my apartment in San Leandro. She was about 75 at that time. She would repeat the same old stories over and over throughout the same day. I remember thinking that would drive me crazy if she were living with me. She had also lost her love of walking. At her place overlooking the ocean in Mexico, she would walk for miles with her little black Scottie. However, she was worn out after a block or two in the city. In her own home, she didn't repeat herself or have problems taking care of her affairs. That is when I realized that she had the same environmental sensitivity problems I have.

As my sensitivity developed, I was not well enough to continue teaching. Instead of Mother coming to live with me, her place became a haven for me. After they retired, my parents had built a home in an American development north of Rosarito on the Baja coast. There was fraud. Lots were sold more than once. The whole thing fell apart. (My parents would want you to know that it was the fault of the American developers.) The

Mexican government stepped in and completed the development down by the ocean, but not the area by the "golf course" where my parents lived. There was no golf course and no utilities. My father had managed to supervise the construction of the house before he died of cancer just two years after retiring. Mother was left with a beautiful home overlooking the Pacific Ocean but no water, gas, or electricity! She had to keep the generator going and chase down the water truck.

Mother welcomed me with open arms. I don't know what I would have done without her. But, of course, we had to make everything chemically clean. I was just as self-centered as other people at level III withdrawal. I turned Mother's whole life upside down. We couldn't use the gas stove, make a fire in the fireplace, or turn on the kerosene heater. I was consulting with Dr. Erlander at this time, and of course, we had to do exactly as he said. That winter was pretty miserable without the fireplace or the kerosene heater. We held glass bottles filled with hot water to try to stay warm. We moved the gas stove outside. I can remember the potatoes turning black before they cooked on windy days.

My diet was basically cabbage and other vegetables in that food family, some kinds of fish, white potatoes, and olive oil. Mother went on these foods with me. When I arrived, Mother was steadily losing weight. She weighed 80 pounds and was about five feet tall. She had been eating virtually a vegetarian diet because she didn't like meat. While living alone, her typical evening meal consisted of a large bowl of millet topped with steamed vegetables and a glass of milk. Millet is a grain closely related to corn. After she had been off of millet for about a year, we decided to try it again. Mother became very ill after eating the millet. After Mother got off the foods she was reacting to, she started to regain weight until she was about 115 pounds. I mention this now because so many elderly people are frail and can't gain weight. The trick is to get off the foods that are causing reactions. After about two years, Mother started getting painful arthritis from reactions to potatoes. We had great difficulty finding safe foods for her from then on. She never became thin again because we tried to remove anything she was reacting to from her diet.

We wanted to get back to the United States, but how were we going to do it with very little money and our need for a clean, unpolluted environment? We began exploring along the US side of the border. We discovered Jacumba. Jacumba is a little town of about 800 people in the far southeast corner of San Diego County and right on the Mexican border. Before air conditioning, people from El Centro and the Imperial Valley Desert had come up the mountain to Jacumba Hot Springs. But, air conditioning had come in, and the freeway had bypassed the town. As a result, property values had sunk to the lowest in the county. Best of all, the mountains blocked the pollution from San Diego and LA.

We were able to buy one of the old summer cottages built in 1930. It had not been lived in for ten years and was in poor repair, but to us it was a treasure. Later we learned that it was built of redwood, so there had never been any mold or termite problems. We had found a place that was safe for us, and I was very much afraid of using any building materials, paint, or chemicals that we might react to. Mother became very sick for several days when we painted the bathroom with regular, white paint. We tried using something called "milk paint," but it acted like a paint stripper. The man we had hired tried valiantly to steam off the mess and put more milk paint on. The walls really looked diseased, but we left them that way. It was much more important to be safe than to be pretty. Except for the walls, it really was a charming cottage.

Mother had her own agenda for leaving her home and coming back to the United States. She wanted to take care of her sister, Elizabeth, who was in a nursing home with Parkinson's disease. Mother had not been able to take Elizabeth down to Mexico for more than three weeks at a time without losing her sister's financial support from the state of California. Aunty Elizabeth had always been very special to her nieces and nephew. She was so sweet and gentle and didn't have children of her own. I'll never forget how happy she was to get in our car and ride home with us from the nursing home.

The story of Elizabeth is another piece of the puzzle, but this chapter is Mother's story. Mother was about 78 years old when we brought Elizabeth home. It took both of us to care for Elizabeth during the last two years of her life. We had no idea what we were getting into. At that time, it was very difficult to care for a Parkinson's patient; she became paralyzed inch by inch. Mother was a great help. She was a care provider and doing very well for her age. However, she could become anxious or depressed if she got ahold of the wrong foods.

One afternoon I found Mother sitting on a pile of clothes out in the washroom crying miserably. I asked her what was wrong. She said that I had said something mean to her and that was why she was crying, but she couldn't remember what I had said. I told her that I hadn't said anything to her. In fact, we hadn't even been together. We tried to figure out what she might have eaten or been exposed to that would make her so depressed. We traced it back to some celery she had eaten. For years after that, I was very careful not to let her have celery.

Mother's health declined noticeably after her 80th birthday, but she was still a big help. I was busy with my small business, Safe Haven, selling reading boxes and nutritional supplements. Paula, who later became our postmaster, was wrapping packages and putting reading boxes together. Mother made lunch for us, usually a big baked potato with lots of sour cream. (For years, I thought I was reacting to grains but not to milk.) She also loved to make cherry pies. Sometimes she played the piano for us. Even after she broke her hip, she recovered surprisingly well and got around with her walker.

By the time Mother was 83, I had to admit that Safe Haven was never going to support us, and I decided to find out if I was well enough to return to teaching. I got a job as a special education teacher at an elementary school in Imperial, which is just north of El Centro. I commuted 50 miles down the mountain and across the desert each way. I was gone at least ten hours a day, but Mother was able to take care of the house and watch our beautiful German shepherd, Susie.

It was not until Mother was 85 that she needed caregivers. She had broken the other hip, and now she didn't want to use the walker. She couldn't remember what she was supposed to do, and I was afraid she might wander away from the house. After she died, we learned that Mother had had Alzheimer's disease, but at the time, we continued to treat her as a person with environmental illness and chemical sensitivity. Dr. Randolph always said that Alzheimer's disease was quite distinct from food and chemical sensitivities. As we will see in the next chapter, there are additional significant factors involved in Alzheimer's disease.[192] If Mother had lived in the city with all the chemical exposures that most Americans face, she would have had Alzheimer's by age 75 or even earlier. By living in a clean environment and being careful of her diet, she had gained ten years of normal life. By continuing this type of care, we were able to prevent some of the worst aspects of the disease. She knew me up to the end. She also knew my brother to the end, although he was only able to come once or twice a year.

It is hard to find the right person to care for an Alzheimer's patient. Some people assume that anyone off the street who will take the minimum wage will do. These patients can be demanding, frustrating, angry, and even violent. What if the caregiver rears back and becomes angry in return? It is so frightening to think that you might leave your beloved parent with someone who is on alcohol or drugs, someone who is mean or even cruel, or someone who might just walk off and leave them before you got home. We were 60 miles away from the outskirts of metropolitan San Diego, which was much too far to use a professional service. I had to find a local person. I was blessed to find Elaine Sanders. She and her husband were caretakers at the American Legion Camp. Elaine is a person of unusual strength, integrity, and empathy for the elderly. I always knew that I could count on her. With Elaine and our trustworthy backup helpers, Mellie and Betty, during the day and me during nights and weekends, we were there for Mother.

Elaine had a regular routine. First, she would help Mother dress. Mother had her own ideas of what she wanted to wear. It had to be red. Her favorite sweater was red with black Scotties. Next came breakfast. Elaine would give her just one food so that we could tell which foods were bad for her. After breakfast, they would have their Spanish lesson. They always started on Lesson One. Mother learned the lesson quickly and felt a real sense of accomplishment. She loved learning, but after half an hour or 45 minutes, she would be tired. The next morning they would start at the beginning of Lesson One again. Then they might sing some fun, easy songs. Mother could remember little jingles from her childhood such as "Farmer in the Dell" and "Twinkle, Twinkle Little Star." Then it was time for a movie and lunch. After lunch, they would walk in the backyard. Sometimes Elaine would just hold her arm. Other times she would use her walker. Finally, Elaine would ask her to play the piano, and they would enjoy the music together.

Elaine treated Mother as her friend and companion and just let herself enjoy entertaining Mother as you would a child. Mother treated Elaine almost like a quest. She could be very charming when company came. Attention was the thing. Mother wanted your total attention. All of this was possible only because we were so careful to avoid chemical exposures and stay away from foods she was reacting to. If we had had a gas stove, if the house had fresh paint on it, or if Elaine had worn scented body care products, Mother would have been too angry or depressed for us to work with.

Mother loved to ride in the car. As soon as I would get home, she wanted to go for a ride. We liked to listen to Garrison Keillor tapes as we drove. Her favorite story was "Rhubarb Pie." She would always tell me about the big rhubarb patch outside her grandmother's back porch. The same stimulus always brought the same response. Every time we passed the Caltrans Yard with its small deodar cedars, she would remind me of Christmas Tree Lane in Altadena. When I was home during the summers, Mother and Susie usually managed to talk me into three rides a day. Mother never remembered that we had just gotten back from a ride, and Susie would bark and look as me with eager eyes. Many times, as we were riding together, Mother told me that this was the happiest time of her life. Of course, she had forgotten other happy times.

Mother liked to watch old movies. We watched VHS tapes on our little black and white television because Mother was very sensitive to electrical waves, EMF radiation. It only took a few minutes of watching a color television to make her feel sick all over. She didn't just watch a movie once or twice, she watched the same movie dozens of time, and she expected you to watch it with her. She wanted your full attention. She didn't want you to sort the mail or clean the house while she watched the movie. This validated the experience. This was something you enjoyed together, not a baby-sitting activity. We must have watched *Random Harvest* with Ronald Colman and Greer Garson and the wartime movie *Mrs. Miniver* 50 or 60 times. I would always fast forward past the scenes in Mrs. Miniver where Greer Garson manages to wrestle the gun away from the wounded German soldier. That small amount of violence was too upsetting to Mother. Even as a much younger woman, she had not been able to handle conflict, especially an emotional upset in the family.

On a good day, Mother could follow and enjoy a full-length movie, but not when she was reacting. One afternoon while we were watching *The Sound of Music*, I gave her a small dish of sherbet. She suddenly said, "Can't we change the page now?" She was unhappy and didn't want to watch the movie because she was reacting to the sherbet. She didn't say "change the movie," or "change the station," but instead she said "change the page." She had a tendency to substitute a word or expression that was close but not quite right for the correct word, such as asking for a "jar" instead of a "bowl." However, your instructions to her had to be absolutely correct. She wouldn't drink out of a "mug" if you had told her to drink out of a "cup." Once while I was pushing her in her wheelchair up a brick path, I asked her to put her feet on the ground. She continued to hold her feet up. When I asked her why, she said that she couldn't put her feet on the ground because the bricks were on top of the ground.

We had some advantages in trying to improve Mother's health. She had never taken prescription drugs; the only medications we used were antibiotics when needed and a nitroglycerin patch at the end. Shortly before I joined her, Mother had arranged to have her back teeth extracted to remove the mercury. She had gold crowns over old amalgam fillings, which is known to be detrimental. If she had not done that, we might not have been able to help her very much. She was also willing to stay on a restricted diet.

Mother's regular doctor was Dr. Almaden, M.D. in Brawly, which was 60 miles away. A caregiver would drive Mother to my school, and I would take her into Brawly for her appointments. We always practiced the doctor's name on the way to his office, but when he would ask her his name, she could never quite remember. She was charming and cheerful for these office visits. Dr. Almaden never put a label on Mother's condition. He helped us with specific problems such as bronchitis or abdominal pain. She had a couple of short stays in Pioneer Memorial Hospital. She was miserable and uncooperative from all the food and chemical exposures in the hospital. However, after getting home, she had no memory of the experience.

Both acupuncture and chiropractic care proved to be very helpful. We took her to a well-known chiropractor in La Jolla, Dr. Randy Crisp, who has since passed away. His adjustments to her back and hips enabled Mother to stay mobile and continue walking with a walker long after most people would have been in a wheelchair. He lifted her mood with cranial manipulation. She was always much happier and more cooperative after he worked with her. After about three months, these benefits would fade, and we would need to make another 75-mile trip into La Jolla.

We went to Dr. Tai-Nan Wang in the Clairmont District for acupuncture. I was always careful to tell Mother several times on the way that we were going in for an acupuncture treatment. However, when we arrived she was always upset because I hadn't warned her. She would be a good sport and let the doctor treat her, but she was impatient. She would count down with the timer loud enough for the doctor to hear. I once asked Dr. Wang if he thought Mother had Alzheimer's. He didn't think so because she had a sense of humor. He said that he had worked with many Alzheimer's patients, and they had no sense of humor. Mother practically floated out of his office, but after several months, we would need to have another treatment. I wish I had a video showing the lift she got from both the chiropractic and acupuncture treatments.

Our biggest frustration was that we couldn't find any "safe" foods for Mother. In a note that I left for a temporary caregiver, I warned that Mother might become dizzy or have a bad coughing spell after eating, or that she might become tired, anxious, demanding, sad, or hyper. My instructions were to write down what she had eaten, to use steam from the teakettle for the cough, and "be patient. It will pass." It is likely that she became a "universal reactor," just as I did, because of a dysfunctional digestive system. She frequently told us that she didn't want any meat, and the age spots on the back of her hands became very heavy and dark. In the end, whipping cream was the only food we could rely on. Her reactions became increasingly strong from temper tantrums to anxiety. She would become confused and forget where her bed was and how to turn on a faucet. When she would get angry, she would threaten to take her oriental carpets and go to her house.

One evening Mother was sitting in the kitchen with me while I prepared my lunch for the next day. When she saw me cutting celery sticks, she asked for a piece. It had been years since she had any raw celery, so I cut an inch from the bottom of the stalk and handed it to her. She said it tasted wonderful, so "fresh" tasting. About half an hour later, while we were watching television in the living room, Mother suddenly turned to me. She had the saddest look I have ever seen on a human face. She looked straight at me and said, "My two children are looking for me. How can they ever find me? They don't know where I am. How can they find me?"

I looked at her and said, "It's the celery!" I tried to comfort her and assure her that everything would be fine, but to her the anxiety and concern over her children who were searching for her was very real. We had to wait about half an hour for the reaction to wear off. Then she knew me.

Sometimes when people try to make the house especially nice for an Alzheimer's patient, they trigger unexpected reactions. One lovely spring afternoon I picked a sprig of lilacs from the large bush in our backyard. Mother had always loved lilacs. I carried it into the house and held it up to her face. She suddenly became very angry. I looked down at my arm sticking out toward her with the lilacs right under her nose and quickly jerked my arm back and removed the flowers from the house. We would have to enjoy the flowers outside in the open air. Mother became calm again as soon as I had removed the lilacs from the house.

Mother was exquisitely sensitive to her bedding. To avoid commercial mattresses with their foam, fire retardants, and other chemicals, we had gotten iron beds with flat springs, the kind you see in Goodwill and Salvation Army thrift shops. On the flat springs, we piled about ten wool blankets (without mothproofing) folded in half. We covered the wool with a heavy cotton spread. Our cotton sheets and blankets went on top of this. This worked very well for me, but Mother reacted even to all natural, organic bedding. I dreaded it when she couldn't sleep because I hated to get up and change her bedding. If I didn't change it, she would be so unhappy and ornery the next morning that it wasn't worth it. It was what actually touched her that was most important. She slept in a heavy, white, cotton sweater (made in Mexico) until it was nothing but a rag. Two close friends sent some beautiful bedding that had been in their families for several generations. Various ways of laundering the blankets had to be tested also. We tried everything from old linen table clothes to yards of rayon and silk fabric. This was almost as difficult as the food problem.

One night I got up at about two in the morning to help Mother to the bathroom. When it was time to take her back to bed, she became stubborn and refused to get up off the toilet. She was too heavy for me to lift without her cooperation. How was I going to get her back to bed? I remembered that a little gadget that I had ordered for acupressure on myself was still sitting in its box on the dining room table. This small tool was widely advertised in the eighties for pain relief and acupressure. Two pieces of metal rubbing together caused a small charge (there were no batteries). I took it out of the box and tried it on the back of my hand. The charge was quite mild, so I took it back to the bathroom. I put it on Mother's temple and clicked it once. She immediately became docile and cooperative. This is something that should be investigated for Alzheimer's patients. I only used it a couple of times because Mother didn't like it.

All electric equipment produces electrical and magnetic fields of different kinds. Our chiropractor, Dr. Crisp, knew that Mother was very sensitive to some electromagnetic fields, EMF. He suggested that we get an appliance that would help organize the electrical fields in the house. We got the whole house unit for Mother and a wristwatch for me. This unit was very helpful. Mother was calmer and less hyper after we got it. She had often been impatient and wanted things to be done instantly. After the unit was plugged in, she was better inside the house. However, she was more sensitive to outside ambient EMF from things such as electrical wires and radio transmissions. One morning, soon after getting this unit, we decided to celebrate Mother's upcoming birthday by driving to Julian, a charming little town in the mountains about an hour and a half away. Mother was looking forward to our adventure. Several miles away from home, Mother started becoming unhappy and anxious. She didn't know why she was unhappy because she wanted to go on the trip. It occurred to me that if this was an EMF problem, my wristwatch might help. I put my watch on her right wrist. (Using kinesiology,

Dr. Crisp had determined that I should wear the watch on my right wrist. He had said that knowing which side of the body to put the watch on was very important.) We drove on for a couple of miles. Mother continued to become more unhappy. I pulled over to the side of the road again and put the wristwatch on Mother's left wrist. This worked. Within minutes, Mother was cheerful and eager for the trip. We had a good day.

In August of 1994, my *Alternatives* health newsletter arrived with information in it that would prove to be very helpful to us. Although he knew that he might be criticized for it, Dr. David Williams had written about amaroli, the practice of drinking one's own urine. For hundreds of years, other cultures have used urine to treat various health problems. Using urine has alleviated conditions from infections, to allergies, to insomnia, and rheumatoid arthritis. In India and China, it is used to promote longevity. Dr. Williams referred to a study done in Carluke, Scotland, in which urine therapy was effective in controlling food and chemical allergies. I went to Mother with this article in some excitement. She said, "You do it first!" After trying it for about a month, I told her that it made a huge difference and urged her to try it. She agreed. It proved to be one of the most helpful things we did. When toileting became difficult, we stopped for a few weeks. Mother declined so rapidly that Elaine and I decided that we would manage to continue.

(*Alternatives* August 1994, Vol. 5, No. 14. For back issues phone 800-718-8293. Dr. Williams doesn't recommend using this therapy for someone who is pregnant or for people who drink or smoke heavily, take prescription or recreational drugs, or have kidney disease. Other cautions are included in the article.)[193] An excellent book on this subject is *Your Own Perfect Medicine* by Martha Christy.[194]

At the end of Jewel Valley Road, there is an open area where the rabbits like to come in the evening. Mother, Susie, and I would sit very quietly in the car and watch the bunnies. I would point out a bunny next to a rock or one almost hidden by a bush. Mother would follow my directions and be able to see it. As time went on, it seemed as though she couldn't follow my directions. I would tell her that there was a bunny close to the car, and she would start looking way out, 50 feet away. Even if I pointed with my arm or took her arm and pointed, she didn't have any idea where to look. It took a while to realize that she was losing her sense of direction. For many years, Mother had had a very poor sense of direction and would almost invariably turn the wrong direction coming out of a restaurant. Toward the end, she no longer knew the location of her own body. It was difficult to get her into bed because she didn't know which way to move her body. If you asked her to move forward a little, she might try to move to one side. Although she had slept on her right side for years, she no longer knew what position to get into after she got in bed.

One afternoon as we were driving toward Jewel Valley Road, Mother started asking me about heaven. I told her that when she reached the pearly gates, she was not going to be able to say she hadn't known what she needed to do in order to get into heaven. I said, "All of your life people have tried to lead you to salvation. You have just been stubborn." To my joy, she responded, "I have been stubborn, and it is true." But then she wondered why after all this time nobody has come back from heaven to tell us about it. I told her there was a place in the Bible that explained that. When we got home, we read the Bible especially the parable of the rich man and Lazarus from Luke 17:19-31. We prayed together, and she accepted Jesus as the Son of God who had died for her sins and risen again. That was wonderful, however I thought to myself that she would not remember, and we would have to do this over and over again. But she was at peace and did not mention the subject again.

My brother, David, played an important part in our lives even though he wasn't able to visit very often. We knew that if we really got into financial trouble or if there was an emergency, we could count on him. He lived with his family in Washington, D.C., and he would come to see us once or twice a year. His visits were always a high point. That was the one time that Mother would let her caregivers leave her side to clean house and get ready. She was always at her best when David came. I am mentioning these visits because it is important to know that Mother did not forget her son even though she did not see him very often. One of the most heart breaking aspects of Alzheimer's is when a beloved parent or spouse no longer recognizes the loved one who is caring for them. When David turned to leave after what would be their last visit, he had tears in his eyes. Mother called him back and held open her arms to hold him tight. (They had both forgotten that Elaine was in the room. She was so touched that she told me about it afterwards.)

Not long after David's visit, Mother sank into a lethargic state. She just slept all the time, maybe 22 out of 24 hours. Sometimes she would be awake, but she wanted to stay in bed. This lasted for several months. It became very difficult to care for her. We did have a wonderful nurse from a hospice. When we could no longer take Mother to her regular doctor in Brawley, we called on a doctor from the rural clinic that would make house calls. He told us that she had Alzheimer's and wanted to know why we hadn't put her in a nursing home. Her caregivers and I were disgusted after all the trouble we had gone to in order to keep her at home. I went to his office and tried to explain to him that she had an immune system problem. To him, Mother had Alzheimer's and that was that.

I began wondering if the condition I was calling "an immune system problem" was what other people called "Alzheimer's." It seemed very important to know. If Mother really had Alzheimer's disease, it would mean that some of the things we had done to help her might help other people with Alzheimer's. I arranged for an autopsy with the San Diego Alzheimer's Association. The results from the Research Pathologist at the Directory, National Alzheimer's Disease Brain Bank & Research came back: "These findings are consistent with a diagnosis of Alzheimer's Disease."

Mother died in her 90th year at home in her own bed. She knew Elaine and me to the very end. She called to me by name twice the last week to ask for a drink of water. She died quietly with a lovely expression on her face, as if she were seeing something very beautiful.

AVOIDING
ALZHEIMER'S DISEASE

THE OBSERVATIONS AND EXPERIENCES OF PEOPLE who care for Alzheimer's patients together with some unexpected conclusions from the Nun Study can help us understand the root cause of this terrible disease. In the previous chapter, we saw that many of the worst symptoms can be avoided or diminished by removing foods and chemicals that cause immune system reactions. Mother was able to have happy experiences, remember her loved ones, and in many ways, be a companion. However, in the end, the disease overwhelmed her. Evidently, there were factors involved that we did not understand. A registered nurse provided another piece of the puzzle. Sally Pacholok, R.N. observed that many elderly patients who appeared to have Alzheimer's disease actually had an undiagnosed B12 deficiency. Mary Newport, M.D. was desperately searching for a way to help her husband, and she found an alternative energy source that can be used by the brain when it can no longer use glucose normally. Finally, David Snowdon, Ph.D., who directed the Nun Study and knew many of the nuns personally, discovered that homocysteine and small strokes play an important role in whether Alzheimer's symptoms are expressed.

In their book, *Could It Be B12?*, Pacholok and Stuart describe symptoms of B12 deficiency that sound very much like common symptoms of Alzheimer's disease. This book was introduced in the chapter on *The Stomach*. For example, depression, memory loss, paranoia, irritability, violent behavior, poor balance, loss of position sense, generalized weakness, loss of appetite, incontinence, and congestive heart failure are all seen in patients with a B12 deficiency. In fact, these authors state "yet preliminary evidence indicates that deficient B12 levels worsen Alzheimer's symptoms, and that B12 deficiency may even play some role in causing the disease."[195] Later in this chapter, we will examine the part that a low vitamin B12 level plays in Alzheimer's disease.

David Snowdon, Ph.D. is an epidemiologist who has specialized in unique populations of religious groups. He had studied aspects of cancer and the Lutheran Brotherhood and the impact of diet and health on Seventh-day Adventists. After several years of effort, he had pulled together a significant project to investigate education and aging among the nuns of the School Sisters of Notre Dame. The project was funded, and he already knew many of the sisters. Thinking of aging led to thoughts of Alzheimer's and then to the possibility of brain autopsy. Fellow professionals warned Snowden that asking for organ donations might jeopardize his whole project because so few people are willing to donate their brain.

Dr. Snowdon recalls the evening in December 1990 when he spoke with the nuns in their large meeting room at the Mankato convent 90 miles southwest of St. Paul. First he talked about the dehumanizing deterioration of Alzheimer's disease and how little was known about its cause. Finally, he told them the sisters who joined the new study would need to take a mental and physical evaluation each year. They would also be asked to donate their brain tissue after they died. When he concluded, there was dead silence. Then he heard whispering in the back of the room. As the talking grew louder there seemed to be an attitude that their brains weren't going to do them much good after they were buried. Then one of the oldest nuns, age 95, Sister Borgia Leuther spoke: "He is asking for our help. How can we say no?" Serious thought and prayer guided the sisters in making the decision to sign, or not sign, the consent form. The word also had to be taken to the other six convents of the School Sisters of Notre Dame. Ultimately, a phenomenal 66%, or 678 of the 1,027 eligible nuns, joined the brain donation program.[196]

David Snowdon, Ph.D. tells us the story of the Nun Study in *Aging with Grace: What the Nun Study Teaches*

Us About Leading Longer, Healthier, and More Meaningful Lives. It is a beautifully written book that anyone interested in Alzheimer's disease will want to read. The sisters are real people with real feelings, and their privacy is carefully protected. We can't help but care about them as we read their stories.

William Markesbery, M.D., director of the Sander-Brown Center on Aging at the University of Kentucky Medical Center in Lexington, conducted the autopsies. He was known as an empathetic, caring doctor who had treated thousands of Alzheimer's patients. He was also a neuropathologist who had conducted autopsies on thousands of Alzheimer's brains. One of the unusual features of the Nun Study is that Dr. Markesbery did the autopsies "blind" without knowing the mental abilities of the patients in advance. Pathologists usually like to know a patient's symptoms before they give an evaluation.[197]

The distinguishing features of an Alzheimer's brain involve the weight of the brain and the quantity and location of beta-amyloid plaques and tangles. A healthy, adult, female brain weighs about two-and-one-third pounds or 1,100 to 1,400 grams. A person who has Alzheimer's usually has a significantly smaller brain because the disease destroys brain tissue. Sometimes there are even gaping spaces in the cerebral cortex. The development and spread of plaques and tangles seen during the autopsy was described based on the Braak scale. On this scale, stage 0 indicates that there are no plaques and tangles or they are very rare. Stages I through VI indicate increasing levels of the plaques and tangles throughout the thinking areas of the brain. One other physical feature proved to be highly significant. These are the small, discolored, pitted structures of dead tissue, or infarcts, which are the scars left behind by small strokes.[198]

Dementia is not an inevitable result of aging. Almost 40% of the nuns who died between the ages of 96 and 100 ranked at I or 0 on the Braak scale, which indicates that some people are relatively resistant to the development of Alzheimer's disease. Sister Borgia Leuther, who had urged the other nuns to join Dr. Snowden's project, had a beautiful brain. When she died at 103 years, her brain did not show any evidence of tangles, Braak scale 0, and there were no signs of strokes.[199]

In most cases, the autopsy reports correlated with the tested abilities of the nuns. As we would expect, the brains of those who were mentally sharp showed almost no evidence of disease, while those who had dementia had obvious signs of damage. There was a close relationship between the Braak stages at autopsy and the mental health of the participants. However, some participants whose brains had only a few plaques and tangles still had the symptoms of Alzheimer's disease. At Braak stages I and II, 22% had these symptoms. At

Braak stages III and IV, 43% had symptoms, and at stages V and VI, 70% had dementia.[200]

These results raised important questions. Why did some participants who were only at Braak I or II already have full-blown Alzheimer's disease? Why didn't 100% of the nuns who were at Braak V or VI, with brains riddled with plaques and tangles, have Alzheimer's? This is where the evidence of strokes becomes important. If small brain infarcts or pits caused by small strokes were found during the autopsy then fewer tangles were required for a person to show signs of dementia. However, if a person had not had any strokes, they might have large numbers of plaques and tangles and yet be intact mentally before they died. Forty-three percent of the nuns who had an "Alzheimer's brain" but didn't show evidence of strokes had not experienced the symptoms of Alzheimer's disease. Strokes appear to act as a "trip switch" in those who already have plaques and tangles in their brains and cause the symptoms to be expressed. According to Dr. Snowdon, "it also strongly suggests that stroke-free brains can compensate for Alzheimer's lesions to some extent and mute the symptoms of the disease."[201]

Vascular health appears to be connected to Alzheimer's disease in another important way. When autopsy results were compared to blood samples, higher levels of folic acid in the blood were found to lessen the chance of brain atrophy. Folic acid along with vitamin B12 keeps homocysteine from building up. If homocysteine reaches unsafe levels it may damage brain cells and increase the atrophy of the Alzheimer's brain. There is a connection between brain atrophy, low folic acid, and high homocysteine.[202] Vitamin B12 was not investigated in the Nun Study. However, other research indicates B12 is more significant than folate in maintaining healthy levels of homocysteine.[203] [204] Those who had vascular damage but did not have plaques and tangles didn't have the classic mental Alzheimer's symptoms. The most serious symptoms were expressed when a person had an "Alzheimer's brain" plus vascular damage.[205]

We owe a profound debt of gratitude to the nuns of the School Sisters of Notre Dame who took part in the Nun Study and to Dr. Snowdon and his colleagues who directed the project with meticulous care and attention to detail. Through them, we gained insights into the causes of Alzheimer's disease, which we could not have learned in any other way.

We now have three pieces of the Alzheimer's puzzle: allergies, in the broad sense as used by clinical ecologists, B12 deficiency, and vascular damage caused, at least in part, by high homocysteine. Allergies, low B12, and high homocysteine levels all stem from inadequate stomach function. Over the age of 60, up to 30% of people have atrophic gastritis or atrophy of the stomach. By the time a person reaches the age of 70, the chance of his having atrophic gastritis is 50%.[206] When the stomach doesn't produce sufficient hydrochloric acid, an over growth of *H. pylori* bacteria can easily develop. In one study, researchers found *H. pylori* antibodies in both the serum and cerebral spinal fluid of patients with Alzheimer's disease. The severity of the patients' dementia correlated with increasing levels of the antibodies. Eradication treatment resulted in improvement in cognitive and functional ability. In another study, 88% of Alzheimer's patients were found to have an *H. pylori* infection.[207] These studies on *H. pylori* bacteria corroborate the evidence that Alzheimer's patients are low in hydrochloric acid and have poor stomach function.

What could cause so many people to have a weak stomach? It could be caused by our high carbohydrate diets because insulin is intimately tied up with acid production.[208] Inflammation from allergic reactions could also damage the parietal cells in the stomach lining. As we discussed in the chapter on the stomach, the question of whether low hydrochloric acid causes allergies or allergies cause low hydrochloric is a chicken-and-egg problem. In many people, the deterioration of the stomach begins as a child perhaps because of a milk or wheat allergy. Inflammation causes parietal cells to die. Less hydrochloric acid is produced. Proteins are not completely digested. The person begins to react to many foods. *H. pylori* bacteria may become established and cause further deterioration of the stomach lining. The stomach becomes dysfunctional, and the immune system reactions become more serious. Research supports the idea that Alzheimer's develops gradually over a person's life. German scientists, Heiko and Eva Braak, who designed the scale used in the Nun Study, autopsied over 800 brains as they searched for patterns in the "Alzheimer's brain." The Braaks estimate that it may require 50 years or longer for the plaques and tangles of Alzheimer's to progress from stage I to stage V or VI, the most serious stages.[209]

According to Joseph Rogers, PhD in *Journal Watch*, which provides expert summaries from 300 medical journals, "chronic, microlocalized brain inflammation is an accepted hallmark of Alzheimer's disease." This inflammation can be tested decades before symptoms of dementia appear. In a major, longitudinal study, the Honolulu-Asia Aging Study, 8,006 Japanese-American men were tested beginning in 1965. Twenty-five years later, 3,734 were screened and carefully examined for dementia. A random subset of 1,000 men had their C-reactive protein concentrations measured from serum taken during the initial testing. C-reactive protein was used to measure inflammation. Those with high markers for inflammation had a three-fold greater risk of dementia. It was concluded that inflammation may be present decades before a person shows signs of dementia.[210]

Alzheimer's develops after a lifetime of reacting to the foods and chemicals in the environment. Most people with this disease started their life at level I stimulus. They were charming and attractive as young people. In middle age, they experienced level II and struggled with weight problems. Then, in their fifties and sixties or sixties and seventies, they entered level III and started losing weight. At first, they were delighted with their new, trim selves. However, they began to experience anxiety, sleep problems, forgetfulness, brain fog, and other mental symptoms. They began to look not just thin but frail. This sets the stage for Alzheimer's disease. This life-pattern corresponds to the pattern of stimulus and withdrawal identified by Theron Randolph, M.D. that has been the focus of this book.

Research tends to support the pattern of weight gain and loss that is part of the Randolph paradigm. That is, a heavy, robust, level II person can morph into a mild, thin level III person and become frail as an older adult. It has been discovered that weight gain and loss can be used as a predictor of Alzheimer's disease. An important study from Kaiser Permanente Division of Research, published in 2008, found that obesity in midlife increased the risk of dementia, including Alzheimer's disease, several decades later. A longitudinal analysis was conducted of 6,583 members of Kaiser Permanente of Northern California who had their belly fat and weight measured when they were between the ages of 40 and 45. Over 30 years later, their medical records were checked to see how many had developed some form of dementia. A total of 1,049 were diagnosed with dementia. Those who had been obese with a big belly had over a threefold chance of having dementia in their seventies compared to those who had had normal weight and low belly fat in their forties.[211] If this study is extended until the participants are in their eighties, a much higher proportion could be expected to show signs of Alzheimer's and other forms of dementia.

Weight gain in middle age increases the likelihood of dementia decades later; however, losing that extra weight and becoming thin as an elderly person makes dementia, including Alzheimer's, statistically even more likely. A distinction must be made between those who experience unintended weight loss and those who lose weight because of a determined health-building program. It is generally recognized that weight loss is a problem for Alzheimer's patients, and there is increasing evidence that this weight loss often precedes the diagnosis of the disease. In a study done by the Alzheimer's disease Research Center, Washington University School of Medicine, a group of 449 older adults was followed for an average of six years. Eventually, 125 individuals developed Alzheimer's type characteristics. As a group, the participants who developed this type of dementia weighed less at the study enrollment than the participants who remained without dementia. Based on the total study, the authors concluded that weight loss might be a preclinical indicator of Alzheimer's disease.[212] A review of the literature done by Luchsinger and Gustafson in 2009 found significant loss of weight may occur decades before dementia becomes apparent.[213] These studies confirm the picture of a thin person at level III withdrawal.

The typical early-stage or pre Alzheimer's patient is a slender, frail woman in her seventies or eighties with thin, white hair who eats very little meat and almost never has red meat. She is also likely to have many age spots and soft fingernails that tear easily. The thin hair and weak fingernails give away her need for hydrochloric acid. The lack of any appetite for meat, especially red meat, is also an indication that the stomach is not functioning well enough to digest protein completely. She has been bravely struggling for years with many unexplained problems brought on by her hidden allergies, and recently she has been coping with anxiety and even depression at level III withdrawal. Now something unfair happens. She can no longer absorb vitamin B12. Her stomach function has become so poor that she does not produce enough hydrochloric acid to separate the B12 from protein. Without that step, B12 is not available to her body.

Without adequate B12, levels of homocysteine will increase. Excess homocysteine is toxic to the vascular system. Brain atrophy and the evidence of small strokes are related to high homocysteine levels. Brain scans of Alzheimer's patients have demonstrated that those with high homocysteine have faster disease progression.[214] From the Nun's Study, we learned that small strokes seem to act as a "trip switch" to turn on the expression of Alzheimer's disease. The autopsies showed that there was a "stunning link" between brain infarcts and dementia, but only if the brain had enough plaques and tangles to qualify as an "Alzheimer's brain." Ninety-three percent of the sisters who had an "Alzheimer's brain" and even one infarct in a critical region of the brain had dementia. However, only 57% of the nuns who had an "Alzheimer's brain" but no strokes had dementia.[215]

It is difficult to determine what Alzheimer's symptoms are caused by allergic reactions and which are caused by a vitamin B12 deficiency because both stem from a dysfunctional stomach and are found in the same patient. Some of the signs that are usually attributed to B12 deficiency are the symptoms that make it so difficult for a family to keep a loved one at home. These include falls caused by poor balance, incontinence, paranoia, irritability, and even violent behavior. Taking B12 may not seem to make a difference because long standing B12 deficiency symptoms are often irreversible, but further damage such as the inability to swallow can often be prevented. The neurological damage done by a lack of B12 is progressive and may be the cause of death in most Alzheimer's patients, usually from a heart attack or congestive heart failure.

The Alzheimer's Association website, www.alz.org, contains an excellent outline of the typical progression of a patient's symptoms, "Stages of Alzheimer's." This framework is based on a system developed by Barry Reisberg, M.D., Clinical Director of the New York University School of Medicine's Silberstein Aging and Dementia Research Center. Stage 7, severe or late-stage Alzheimer's disease, is the last stage. At this stage, individuals frequently lose their ability to recognize speech. They need help with eating and toileting. Finally, "individuals lose the ability to walk without assistance, then the ability to sit without support, the ability to smile, and the ability to hold their head up. Reflexes become abnormal and the muscles grow rigid. Swallowing is impaired."[216] Except for the inability to recognize language, these sound like possible symptoms of a B12 deficiency.[217]

If you are trying to avoid Alzheimer's or you are concerned about someone who already has the disease, the first and easiest step is to make sure that vitamin B12 levels are adequate. Both the shots and sublingual tablets are usually effective depending on your circumstances. This should be discussed with your doctor. Taking B12 is extremely safe except for people who have a rare disorder called Leber's hereditary optic neuropathy. These people should never take cyanocobalamin, but there are other forms of B12 they can use.[218] According to Dr. Jonathan Wright, the only way you can take too much vitamin B12 is to fill your bathtub with B12 and drown in it.[219] One of the problems has been that the threshold for a normal serum B12 test is too low. A person might have been tested, told they were in the normal range, and yet still have inadequate B12 levels. If the threshold were raised from 200 pg/ml to 450 pg/ml, many more cases of B12 deficiency would be caught.[220] For everything you need to know about vitamin B12, read *Could It Be B12?* by Sally Pacholok, R.N. and Jeffrey Stuart, D.O.

Regulating vitamin B12 is the easy part. The hard part of caring for an Alzheimer's patient is controlling the allergic reactions. Here again, this is "allergy" in the broad sense as used by clinical ecologists. Alzheimer's disease comes at the end of a lifetime of struggling with allergies. At levels I and II, a person experiences physical reactions such as hay fever, headaches, and heart problems. However, symptoms become mental at levels III and IV. Remember, when Mother ate celery at level III she became depressed and started crying. However, when she was well into Alzheimer's, level IV, and ate celery, she suddenly didn't know me, didn't know where she was, and was despondent that her children wouldn't be able to find her.

It is heartening to see how much progress can be made when both B12 and allergies are controlled. The website of Ronald Hoffman, M.D. contains the case study of E.K., which demonstrates the power of this approach. Dr. Hoffman is a past president of the country's largest organization of complementary and alternative doctors, the American College for Advancement in Medicine (ACAM). He is also a fellow of the American Academy of Environmental Medicine and is a Certified Nutrition Specialist of the American College of Nutrition (ACN). He is the founder and medical director of the Hoffman Center in New York City.[221]

On his website, Dr. Hoffman comments that hidden food intolerance may play a part in Alzheimer's disease. He refers to a study in which gluten sensitive individuals demonstrated a tenfold increase in neurological dysfunction or dementia compared to those individuals who were not gluten-sensitive. Most of these gluten-sensitive individuals did not have the classic intestinal signs of celiac disease.[222]

E.K. began showing signs of Alzheimer's disease at age 73. She became increasingly forgetful and often cried in the morning. Her parents had died, but she believed they were still alive. She became suspicious of her family and began hiding her things. She started getting lost if she went out by herself. When she was left alone, she would panic and start calling out the windows that she needed help. Over a three-year period, her memory loss became profound and she began to forget members of her own family. A serum B12 test was 280 pg/ml, which was considered to be in the normal range. She was started on a prescription drug with little effect.[223]

E.K. was first seen at the Hoffman Center at the age of 76. She still knew her own name, but she no longer knew her location or the date. She was suspicious and uncooperative. Both her homocysteine and methylmalonic acid were elevated. These are both indicators of a B12 deficiency. She was given a series of B12 shots three times weekly for two weeks followed by monthly injections. Dr. Hoffman noted "the apparent efficacy of B12 shots, despite a normal B12 test." She was put on a gluten-free diet. She was also placed on a regimen of nutritional supplements. A list of these supplements together with commentary by Dr. Hoffman is available on his website, www.drhoffman.com.[224]

E.K. gradually improved in memory and mood. Her family reported that she was calmer and could be left alone. Her ability to name objects returned. Episodes of anger, paranoia, and obstinacy occurred less often. She was able to dress, bathe, and eat with minimal assistance. After two years, her improvement was so obvious that her neurologist noted in his insurance report that she had recovered significant memory and shown substantial improvement in the activities of daily living.[225] He concluded:

> There is no evidence of alteration of sleep-wake cycle, mood changes, agitation, wandering, or other affective or personality disorders. She has reached a stable plateau in her neurological state with no evidence of progressive deterioration. I would presently classify her as having minimal dementia in the order of Age Related Memory Loss.[226]

It is surprising E.K. could make so much progress by just eliminating gluten grains along with B12 injections and nutritional supplements. At least in my limited experience, most individuals with food intolerance react to many foods. If caregivers try to eliminate foods that seem to make a much-loved patient worse, they have to feed her something else. After a few meals, the patient starts reacting to the new food. Finally, the caregivers can't find any safe foods and every food seems to make the patient worse. At the same time, a B12 deficiency causes insidious, progressive neurological damage. Ironically, researchers who thought Alzheimer's disease was caused by a B12 deficiency were defeated when cognitive and emotional symptoms caused by allergic reactions didn't disappear when B12 injections were given. Individuals who tried elimination diets were ultimately defeated by the gradual deterioration caused by a B12 deficiency. The characteristic patterns of symptoms in Alzheimer's disease make sense when we realize that both the allergies and the B12 deficiency stem from the atrophy of the parietal cells in the stomach.

Some doctors have been quietly helping their dementia patients with vitamin B12 injections. John V. Dommisse, M.D. is a nutritional physician and psychiatrist (Canadian-board-certified) who practices in Tucson, AZ. He has been studying vitamin B12 since 1976. He cared enough to write a five star review on Amazon for the outstanding book, *Could It Be B12?* He wrote that in the 26 years he has been investigating B12, "NO patient" with memory problems typical of early Alzheimer's went on to Alzheimer's dementia. He was also able to help people with depression and bipolar illnesses. He attributes his success to "permanent optimization of every patient's serum B12 level."[227]

When we first learn many symptoms of Alzheimer's disease can be prevented or diminished, we are full of hope that we can find the magic supplement. The great frustration is that many Alzheimer's patients are virtually universal reactors. Supplements may be just one more thing that causes reactions. However, that is not always the case. Note the success that Dr. Hoffman had with E.K. I have personally found minerals, fats such as omega-3 fish oils, and probiotics are the most likely to be safe.

If we take another look at our typical elderly woman with Alzheimer's disease, we will see that in addition to her hair being thin, she has a high forehead due to a receding hairline. The outside ends of her eyebrows have disappeared, and in some cases there is very little eyebrow left. Her hair and skin are dry. She has trouble staying warm and always wants the heat turned up. These are all signs of low thyroid function. Low thyroid function is usually caused by a deficiency of iodine. If the body is deficient in iodine then the immune system, all of the glands such as the adrenal glands, and the entire endocrine system will be affected. To understand this aspect of the problem read *Iodine: Why You Need It, Why You Can't Live Without It* by David Brownstein.[228] It could well be that our epidemic of iodine deficiency is feeding into our epidemic of Alzheimer's disease.

We learned from the Nun Study that it is essential to prevent small strokes and other vascular damage. When my husband was told recently that he had had a "silent heart attack," he was motivated to read widely about vascular disease. The best book he found was *Reverse Heart Disease Now: Stop Deadly Cardiovascular Plaque Before It's Too Late* by Stephen Sinatra, M.D. and James Roberts, M.D. My husband was so impressed by the book that he bought 20 copies to give to all his friends who have stents or are thinking about getting one. The focus of this book is on natural healing. A health program to prevent Alzheimer's disease should include a strategy for maintaining a healthy cardiovascular system.

Alzheimer's patients are fragile. They are chemically sensitive as well as food sensitive. They can be reacting so much to chemicals that even eliminating many foods might not bring much improvement. Fragrances are one of the worst offenders. Scented candles (even if they are not lighted), incense, and scented cleaning products can overwhelm a chemically sensitive person. Laundry detergent with lovely lemon and lavender fragrance can be especially bad because it gets into the clothing and bedding right next to the skin. Caregivers must use unscented body care products. Watch out for new carpets, fresh paint, and particleboard in closets and furniture. An electric cook-top should be used instead of a gas stove. Notice in the preceding chapter how we tried to protect Mother from chemicals. *Less-Toxic Alternatives* by Carolyn Gorman is an excellent guide to reducing chemical exposures.[229]

If you are concerned about prevention, or if you are caring for an Alzheimer's patient, talk with your doctor about allergy testing and elimination diets. Carefully study the chapter in this book on testing for allergies. If you do decide to eliminate certain foods, don't rush. There is no need to have a test meal at the end of four or five days. That could provoke a bad reaction. If it is obvious that the person you are caring for is better when a food is removed, there is no need to reintroduce the food. You will be encouraged by how much improvement can be achieved by just removing a few foods.

When searching for foods to feed a person who seems to be reacting to everything, start with foods from the bottom of the addiction pyramid. Remember fats and oils are the least likely foods to cause reactions. Fats are digested differently than most foods. Even if the stomach is hardly functioning, fats can sneak through to be broken down by bile. The liver then produces ketones that can be used as energy by the body, especially the brain. There are two ways that a high fat/low carbohydrate diet can be useful. First, an increase in ketones can supply an alternative energy source for the brain if the normal glucose metabolism has been disrupted. Second, fat may also be a "safe food" for a patient who has serious reactions to virtually all the sugars, starches, and proteins. Members of the cabbage family such as organic broccoli, cauliflower, and cabbage are probably the safest vegetables to try. Protein is essential for survival. If you can't find a "safe" protein, it may be that you are dealing with a "universal reactor" who needs probiotic supplements to reestablish the intestinal flora. See the discussion of universal reactors in the chapter titled "The Diet."

There has been great interest in using medium-chain fatty acids to increase the supply of ketones to the brains of Alzheimer's patients ever since Mary Newport, M.D. had success using coconut oil for her husband, Steve. Dr. Newport is the director of neonatology at Spring

Hill Regional Hospital in Florida. She tried giving her husband six to seven tablespoons of coconut oil per day mixed into his food. More than that gave him diarrhea. "He said it was like someone had turned on a light bulb," Mary Newport said. "He was alert, smiling, joking. He was Steve again. He was back." Steve was able to read again, volunteer at his wife's hospital, and mow the lawn. After hearing this story, other caregivers started using coconut oil. Some used it in coffee. Others put it on oatmeal. Not every patient improved, but some did. Mary Hurst, an 83-year-old woman, started dressing herself again. Her daughter said that before the oil, her mother would just sit in the chair all day incommunicative "like a vegetable," without ever getting out of her nightgown and robe. Mary Hurst even remembered where her birthday cake had been put the day before and opened the refrigerator door.[230]

The results of her experiment with coconut oil have been so impressive that Dr. Newport has written a book, *Alzheimer's Disease: What if There Was a Cure? The Story of Ketones.* Mary Newport shares with us the personal trauma of her husband's descent into Alzheimer's disease and the heartbreak of being turned down for clinical trials for people with mild to moderate Alzheimer's disease because Steve didn't score high enough on the Mini-Mental Status Exam. Soon after this experience, Dr. Newport made a chance discovery that turned their lives around. While she was on the Internet investigating clinical trials, she stumbled on a press release from Accera, a small biotech firm working toward Food and Drug Administration approval. Accera reported that AC1202 actually improved memory in a significant number of people with Alzheimer's disease.

This is where Mary Newport, the doctor, took over. She was curious about how this drug could improve memory since, at present, the FDA-approved drugs for Alzheimer's disease only claim to slow the progress of the disease at best. Discussion on the patent application reviewed information concerning nerve cells in certain parts of the brain that are not able to use glucose normally for energy and eventually die. This same problem with glucose happens in other neurodegenerative diseases such as Parkinson's disease, Huntington's disease, and Lou Gehrig's disease (ALS) but in different areas of the brain. Fortunately, the body has a back-up fuel source. If ketones are available in the bloodstream, they can pass through the blood-brain barrier and provide fuel for neurons and other brain cells. This prospective drug, which was designed to increase ketone levels, was not yet available to the public, but the ingredients were given. Much to Mary's surprise, the main ingredient was medium-chain triglycerides (MCTs) derived from coconuts. (This drug from Accera is now on the market under the name Axona.) [231]

After she finished reading the application, Mary went on an "Internet frenzy" searching for everything she could find about medium-chain fatty acids, coconut oil, MCT oil, and ketones. She learned that coconut oil is nearly 60% medium-chain fatty acids. She calculated that a little over two tablespoons of coconut oil would be an appropriate "dose." The next day, on their way home from yet another mental screening, they stopped at a health food store and bought a quart of coconut oil. The next morning, Mary added two tablespoons of coconut oil to Steve's oatmeal plus a little extra for good measure. Then they got in the car and headed for another testing situation. Much to their delight, Steve scored an 18. This was four points higher than the previous day and six points higher than an earlier test. This was a substantial improvement. Mary had read that some people improve on the first dose, but she was afraid to hope. By the third day of consuming coconut oil, Steve was alert, smiling, and feeling happy when he came into the kitchen for breakfast. He became more animated and talkative and could carry on a conversation. After ten days, Steve even read part of a magazine and began doing gardening chores.[232]

It was three years before Mary Newport wrote about their experiences with ketone therapy. During this time, Steve continued to hold his own and even made progress despite some setbacks. His gait became normal, and he was even able to run. He was no longer depressed and was less distractible. He recognized family members on infrequent visits and could carry on a meaningful conversation. His personality brightened, and his sense of humor returned. There were two days when Steve didn't get his dose of coconut oil in the morning. On both occasions, his Alzheimer's symptoms of confusion and tremors returned until he was given some coconut oil. In 2010, Steve had an MRI to monitor brain atrophy. Between 2004 and 2008 there had been marked atrophy or shrinkage. However, in the MRI done in 2010 his brain was considered stable. It was much more likely the atrophy would have continued to progress. This result was quite surprising and an indication medium-chain fatty acids and ketones were keeping his brain cells alive.[233]

The book by Dr. Newport is full of information. She gives us details of her husband's progress and tells us of her efforts to get the word out to doctors and patients. (Her reception by the Alzheimer's Association was classic!) She explains how ketones work, the history of the ketogenic diet, and important research being conducted by leading scientists. Finally, she reports on the need for funding and the current status of ketone ester, a product that has been developed to increase the availability of ketones to the brain.[234] Frank Shallenberger, M.D. provides helpful information on how he uses ketone therapy with his Alzheimer's patients. He says that although not everyone will benefit as much as Steve did, "in my experience there will always be some degree of improvement." His article, "How to Reverse Alzheimer's Disease," can be found in Dr. Shallenberger's *Real Cures Healing Series, Volume 1*.[235] Bruce Fife, N.D. was the first one to popularize the health-giving benefits of coconut oil. His book, *Stop Alzheimer's Now*, is another good source of information on ketone therapy. Dr. Fife's books *Coconut Lovers Cookbook* and *Coconut Cures* are also helpful.

I now realize that my mother benefited from ketone therapy. In my mother's case, we relied on heavy whipping cream as her primary food for several years because that seemed to be the only food that didn't cause reactions. Since she was getting her calories from cream, we were not forced to feed her other foods that were causing serious reactions such as anger, depression, and memory loss. This was essentially a high fat/low carbohydrate diet, which is a ketogenic diet. According to Dr. Newport, heavy whipping cream contains ketones.[236] Mother undoubtedly benefited from the ketones that are used as brain fuel on this type of diet. When doctors worry about the possible dangers of increasing ketone levels, they are thinking about diabetic ketoacidosis. According to Dr. Newport, the levels of ketones are 50 times higher in diabetic ketoacidosis than after eating a large amount of medium-chain triglyceride oil (20 grams

MCT oil).[237] However, anyone with diabetes, especially type 1 diabetes, needs to work closely with his doctor before going on a diet that will increase ketone levels. Anyone on medications also needs to discuss changes in his diet with his doctor.

We now have four pieces of the Alzheimer's puzzle:

1. Allergies in the broad sense as used by clinical ecologists

2. An inability of neurons and other brain cells to use glucose normally for energy

3. Small strokes

4. A B12 deficiency

With Mother, we were able to cope with two of these dangers. She did not experience the worst symptoms of Alzheimer's disease because we avoided foods and chemicals she was reacting to and also supplied ketones, which her brain cells could use for energy. However, she did have small strokes, and the progressive nerve damage from her B12 deficiency moved forward inexorably. I did not become aware of the part that B12 deficiency plays in Alzheimer's disease until long after Mother had died. The B12 deficiency forces the relentless downward spiral that inevitably leads to death in Alzheimer's disease.

If you are concerned about preventing Alzheimer's disease, forget crossword puzzles! If you think crossword puzzles will protect you from Alzheimer's disease, remember Mother and the Spanish lessons. Be sure you are taking enough vitamin B12. Use coconut oil. I have personally found that taking a couple of tablespoons of coconut oil per day has helped with mental energy and reduced "senior moments." Fight the allergy-addiction battle as best you can. We all know we are eating things we shouldn't. Just taking the B12 and using coconut oil can make a big difference. However, if your health is still poor after you have done those two things, and your doctor can't find a problem, take your allergies seriously. If you are a caregiver, use the simple, basic ideas discussed in this book to improve the quality of life of the person you are helping.

We have felt so helpless in the face of Alzheimer's disease. With over half of people having symptoms of this disease by the time they reach the age of 85, the possibility of this happening to us is all too real. To think of losing our essence, our mind, our personality, and even the memory of our loved ones is too much to face. Now that the causes of this terrible disease are emerging, there are practical solutions. Read this chapter again and think how you can help yourself. Now think how you can help someone you love.

RECOVERY

IN THE 21ST CENTURY, WE ARE FACED WITH AN aging population that is not just old but is also sick. Dementia, cancer, and heart disease are dreaded threats among the elderly. Younger people are faced with diabetes, cancer, and crippling autoimmune diseases, such as rheumatoid arthritis. Even many children require lifelong care from conditions such as autism and developmental disorders. These degenerative conditions drag on year after year and, for younger people, decade after decade. Where did we go wrong? Why did our "Human Experiment" fail?

There must be some basic reasons for this failure because the health of virtually every group that has transitioned from natural, traditional food to the diet of Western civilization has degenerated. Let's take another look at some groups that made this transition. Weston Price was not the only one to witness the decline among groups that abandoned their native diets. There is a rich record of eyewitness accounts left by missionary and colonial doctors. Gary Taubes, in his book *Good Calories, Bad Calories,* has gathered thought-provoking information on the lifestyles, food, and health of many groups before and after they transitioned to a Western diet. The information comes from missionary and colonial physicians, anthropologists, government surveys, and other contemporary evidence.

In 1902, British physician Samuel Hutton began treating patients at a Moravian mission on the northern coast of Labrador. He observed that Eskimos were meat eaters and ate very little plant matter. He found that among those who maintained their traditional diet, European diseases were remarkably rare. "The most striking is cancer," wrote Hutton. Based on 11 years of working in Labrador, "I have not seen or heard of a case of malignant growth in an Eskimo." He also mentioned the absence of asthma and appendicitis. Some Eskimos living near the European settlers had started eating tea, bread, ship's biscuits, molasses, and salt fish or pork. Dr. Hutton observed that these Eskimos were "less robust" and "their children are puny and feeble."[238]

In 1908, the Smithsonian published the first significant report on the health of Native Americans, *Physiological and Medical Observations Among the Indians of Southwestern United States and Northern Mexico*. Ales Hrdlicka,* a physician who also became an anthropologist, wrote this 460-page report after taking six expeditions to

Ales Hrdlicka served for three decades as the curator of the Division of Physical Anthropology at the National Museum in Washington, which is now the Smithsonian's National Museum of Natural History.

the Southwest. He found that malignant disease must be extremely rare among Native Americans. He had not seen "unequivocal signs of a malignant growth on an Indian bone." He noted that among the 2,000 plus Native Americans he examined, he had not seen "one pronounced instance of advanced arterial sclerosis." Varicose veins, hemorrhoids, appendicitis, peritonitis, stomach ulcers, and liver disease were also rare. Dr. Hrdlicka also dealt with the suggestion that Native Americans didn't have chronic diseases because their life expectancy was short. He observed Native Americans lived as long or longer than the local whites.[239]

Other doctors working for the Indian Affairs Bureau also observed that cancer was very rare among Native Americans. For example, Charles Buchannan who practiced medicine for 15 years among 2,000 Native Americans saw only one case of cancer. Henry Goodrich, who provided medical care for 3,500 Native Americans for 13 years, did not see a single case of cancer.[240]

In the United States, the number of cancer deaths rose rapidly in the latter part of the 19th century. In New York, the increase was from 32 per 1,000 deaths in 1864 to 67 in 1900; in Philadelphia, it was from 31 per 1,000 deaths in 1861 to 70 in 1904.[241] The rise was even more dramatic in the 20th century. Now one in two men and one in three women get cancer in their lifetime, and one in four die from cancer despite the miracles of modern medicine.[242]

White flour and sugar were luxury items too expensive for the average person to consume until the middle of the 19th century. However, with the invention of the roller mill and the spread of sugar-beet cultivation, their use rapidly increased. In the United States, the average person used less than 15 pounds of sugar per person per year in the 1830s. By the 1920s, 100 pounds of sugar were being used per person per year. By the end of the last century, the number was up to 150 pounds of sugar per person including high-fructose corn syrup.[243] This does not take into account the great increase in refined carbohydrates, which are broken down as sugar during digestion.[244]

Until the 1970s, most investigators attributed cancer, diabetes, and other diseases of civilization to the increased consumption of refined carbohydrates. First, they blamed the refining process, which stripped starches and sugars of their vitamins, minerals, and fiber. Later they found increased insulin and insulin resistance was responsible for most degenerative diseases. However, by the early 1970s, concern was growing over cholesterol and the role that increased fat consumption plays in heart disease. Doctors began telling their patients to avoid fats, which led to an increase in carbohydrate intake. By that time, much of the research on carbohydrates and the diseases of civilization had been forgotten or was ignored.[245]

Good Calories, Bad Calories: Fats, Carbs, and the Controversial Science of Diet and Health by Gary Taubes is an outstanding and exceptional book. Taubes asks the question "what constitutes a healthy diet?" He searches for a definitive answer to the role that fats and carbohydrates play in the increase in degenerative diseases in our society. He uses historical archives, congressional hearings, laboratory research, books, and interviews to pull together two centuries of nutritional research. After more than 450 pages, he concludes that "dietary fat, whether saturated or not, is not a cause of obesity, heart disease, or any other chronic disease of civilization." He also finds the carbohydrates in the diet, and their effect on insulin secretion, are the problem.[246] Taubes' balanced, in-depth analysis brings authority to his work.

We now know many of the basic mechanisms that cause increased carbohydrate consumption to bring about the degenerative health condition of Western civilization such as diabetes, heart disease, cancer, and obesity. For example, we know that eating sugar requires the pancreas to produce insulin in order to keep blood sugar under control. The more sugar and starches eaten, the more insulin is produced. The cells become insulin resistant and require more and more insulin. The pancreas can no longer keep up with the demand, or the cells no longer respond to the message from insulin.

Blood sugar rises out of control and a person has diabetes. A brief explanation of the mechanisms of some serious conditions is given here to demonstrate how it is possible for the consumption of sugar and refined carbohydrates to cause so much damage. Not all of these hypotheses have been scientifically proven and some aspects are still controversial. For more detailed information, including research and scientific controversies, see an article written by Gary Taubes for the New York Times Magazine, "Is Sugar Toxic?"[247]

Heart disease is closely related to diabetes. Metabolic syndrome, or insulin-resistance, is a major risk factor for both heart disease and diabetes. Chronically elevated insulin levels lead to higher levels of triglycerides and higher blood pressure. It also leads to lower levels of HDL cholesterol, the "good cholesterol."[248] The relationship between a high carbohydrate diet and low HDL cholesterol levels is so reliable that researchers use it to determine the amount of carbohydrates their clinical-trial subjects eat.[249]

Hypertension is one of the diseases of civilization. The average blood pressure in groups eating traditional diets was almost always low. Now we know that increased levels of insulin cause the kidneys to reabsorb sodium rather than excrete it. This causes water retention and higher blood pressure. Insulin also causes the walls of the arteries to thicken and become stiffer. At the same time, the volume within the arteries is decreased. This means that the heart has to push harder to get the blood through the narrowed, more ridged arteries.[250] [251]

One of the most striking advantages of the traditional, non-Western diet is that it does not cause cancer. How can that be? The secret is that cancer cells require sugar to proliferate. Insulin also provides fuel and growth signals to cancer cells by increasing insulin-like growth factor (IGF). Both insulin and insulin-like growth factor will signal otherwise benign tumors to metastasize and migrate. As we age, it is natural for cancerous cells and benign tumors to develop because of genetic errors. What is not natural is for these cells to rapidly multiply and become malignant growths.[252] Our modern diets high in sugars and refined starches lead to chronically high insulin levels. Cancerous cells are virtually bathed in "starter fluid."

High insulin levels also contribute to aging. Cynthia Kenyon, Ph.D., University of California San Francisco, studied mutations that prolong longevity in worms. After she discovered insulin seemed to be involved, she wondered what would happen if she fed glucose to the worms. She added two percent glucose to the medium where the worms lived. The lifespan of the worms was reduced by 25%. When Dr. Kenyon realized that glucose shortened the lives of her worms, she went on a restricted carbohydrate diet. She reported that she lost 30 pounds, her blood pressure, triglycerides, and blood-sugar levels all dropped, and her HDL, the "good cholesterol," increased.[253]

We will end this section on the consequences of a high carbohydrate diet by looking at weight gain. Contemporary observers have frequently reported that those on a traditional diet were lean and strong with great physiques. However, they noted that members of the group who went into the towns and ate European food started gaining weight and often became fat. A fascinating example of this transition happened when the Polynesian islanders of Tokelau migrated to New Zealand. The atolls of Tokelau lie 300 miles south of Samoa, which is so far off the trade routes that they remained isolated until recent times. Until trade routes were opened, the islanders thrived on a diet of coconuts, fish, and breadfruit, which is a starchy melon. More than 70% of their calories came from coconut. Their calories were more than 50% fat and 90% of that fat was saturated.[254]

By the 1960s, New Zealand became concerned about overpopulation of the atolls and instituted a voluntary migration program. More than half of the Tokelauans moved to the mainland. One of the first things they did was to change their diet. Bread and potatoes were eaten instead of breadfruit. Meat replaced fish, and coconuts almost completely disappeared from their diets. Fat consumption dropped and was replaced by sugars and starches. Along with this was an "almost immediate increase in weight." For some, obesity became a problem. This weight gain occurred despite the increased exercise they got by taking jobs as laborers and walking long distances.[255] When the Tokelauans increased their sugars and starches, they also increased their insulin. Insulin doesn't just regulate blood sugar levels; it is also the main regulator of fat metabolism. It signals the cells to burn glucose rather than fat. It also traps the fat in the fat cells by suppressing the enzyme glucagon that enables the fatty acids to slip out of the fat cells so they can be used as energy. It only takes a little extra insulin to suppress this enzyme. Insulin works in a number of ways to store fat. It is only when insulin levels come down that we can use our stored fat for fuel.[256 257]

There must be more to this story. Why do we think an increase in insulin explains all of the degenerative diseases of Western civilization? What about autoimmune diseases, autism, anorexia, depression, attention deficit disorder, schizophrenia, and Alzheimer's disease? A century ago, missionary and colonial physicians never observed these conditions. All of these conditions are caused at least in part by allergies and food intolerance. (Google any of these diseases together with the word *allergies* and see how many results you get.) We discovered this was true in Alzheimer's disease. Could it be that there are a number of serious conditions in which the mechanisms involved are similar to those found in Alzheimer's disease? An increase in insulin causes a decrease in stomach acidity.[258] Could a weakened stomach bring on allergies, B12 deficiency symptoms, and high homocysteine levels in various combinations in different people?

In a professional review, doctors at Zurich University Hospital, Zurich, Switzerland, reported that about 400 million people worldwide have neurological and mental disorders. Neuropsychiatric diseases such as Alzheimer's disease, Parkinson's, depression, and stroke account for about 35% of the total burden of disease in Europe. The annual cost of care for these diseases exceeds those of cancer, cardiovascular conditions, and diabetes in Europe.[259] In 2011, the European College of Neuropsychopharmacology published a three-year study of 30 European countries, which showed an "exceedingly high burden" of neuropsychiatric disorders. About 100 conditions were considered, including depression, addictions, anxiety, schizophrenia, multiple sclerosis, and Parkinson's disease. Another major study in 2005 found that 27% of the adult European Union population had mental illnesses.[260]

Neuropsychiatic disorders are also increasing in the United States, an article in the February 2008 Scientific American reported that almost one out of ten adults in

America is now taking drugs to combat depression.[261] Roughly one out of every four women between the ages of 40 and 59 are taking antidepressants.[262] Mood disorders appear to be increasing. Each successive generation of individuals born since World War II seems to have a higher incidence and earlier age of onset of both major depression and bipolar disorder.[263]

There has been great interest in the genetic causes of neuropsychiatric diseases such as genetic variants of MTHFR and homocysteine metabolism, T allele and cerebro-vascular disease, and APOE-4 and Alzheimer's disease. It is true that these conditions tend to run in families. Our genes may explain why an individual gets one disease rather than another. However, if we go back far enough on the family tree, we will find that our ancestors, who passed these genes on to us, did not have neuropsychiatric diseases.

Words like "neuropsychiatric" sound sophisticated, scientific, and unfathomable, but let's go back to something basic: the stomach. One doctor took a particular interest in how the stomach was affected by the transition from a traditional diet to the diet of Western civilization. Surgeon Captain T. L. Cleave was a physician of the British Royal Navy. He ended his career directing medical research at the Institute of Naval Medicine. Cleave corresponded with hundreds of physicians around the world by requesting information on disease rates in specific situations. He is known for his book, *The Saccharine Disease,* on the dangers of sugar, but in 1962, he also wrote *Peptic Ulcer.* This book provides evidence of the weakening of the stomach when traditional diets were abandoned. In group after group, ulcers were virtually unknown until the people started eating sugar, refined flour, and white rice. For example, in Ethiopia, the staple food of the peasants living in the country was unrefined teff, a grain related to millet. Their consumption of sugar was negligible. Among these peasants, peptic ulcer was rare. However, in the large towns of Ethiopia, such as Addis Ababa, there were bakeries producing white bread and sweets. In these towns, peptic ulcers were common.[264]

Cleave believed ulcers were caused because refined carbohydrates lacked the protein necessary to buffer the gastric acid in the stomach. This is not correct. We now know the *H. pylori* bacteria causes ulcers. However, when people were on their traditional diets, their stomachs were strong and produced lots of hydrochloric acid. This prevented an overgrowth of the *H. pylori* bacteria. It was only after the stomach had weakened that the *H. pylori* bacteria could do its damage. This is why Cleave's observation that peptic ulcers occurred only after people had transitioned to a Westernized diet is significant.

Cleave also studied the normal ranges of gastric acidity in men and women of different ages. His findings were based on an analysis of 3,746 patient records at the Mayo clinic. Stomach acidity is very low in infancy and climbs steadily as children age. In the adult, the amount of acidity continues to increase until about the age of 30. It reaches "a considerably higher level" in men than in women. However, in old age the amount of acidity declines, especially in men, so after the age of 70 it is about the same in both men and women.[265]

The fact that men tend to have more stomach acid than women helps to answer a question that has bothered me for years. Why do so many more women than men have diseases like Alzheimer's, autoimmune diseases, and environmental illness? When I used to get together with a few EI (environmental illness) friends, we would ask each other "where are the men?" We had heard there were seven women for every man with EI. If health problems that involve allergies and food intolerance are initiated by inadequate hydrochloric acid, women will naturally be more susceptible.

Women are also more vulnerable to certain disease states because they require more iodine than men require. Every cell in the body requires iodine, but the greatest concentrations are in the thyroid and reproductive organs. In women, the need for iodine in the breasts and ovaries means they require more iodine than men require. Iodine levels have fallen 50% in the United States in the last 30 years. When the body does not have adequate levels of iodine, the thyroid gland takes the lion's share of what is available. That means other tissues of the body may have severe deficiencies. This could include the immune system, breast tissue, the brain, and the gastrointestinal tract.[266] Many organs need iodine but can't absorb it until the blood measurements reach very high levels. Iodine increases the acidity of the stomach, but the stomach can't take in iodine in significant amounts until the blood level reaches 100 times what the thyroid needs.[267] According to David Brownstein, M.D., "in an iodine deficient state, a woman will show earlier signs and more severe signs of iodine deficiency than a man in a similar deficient state."[268] Insufficient levels of hydrochloric acid and iodine could explain why most neuropsychiatric illnesses are much more common in women than in men.

Randolph's paradigm of stimulus and withdrawal helped us understand the way Alzheimer's develops. It can also help us understand other conditions involving the immune system. Dr. Randolph wrote that he had treated about 20,000 patients for food allergies and related problems. He estimated about 7,500 of these people were suffering primarily from so-called "mental" problems. Most of these patients improved significantly, often after conventional medicine had failed.[269]

Dr. Randolph's major work was published in 1980, but in an interview published in *The Human Ecologist* during the fall of 1991, he said, "I knew what I needed to know by 1960."[270] This would mean that the patients he was seeing were born at the end of the 19th century and the beginning of the 20th century. The sisters who participated in the Nun Study were also born at the turn of the century. My mother was born in 1907. Think how much we have deteriorated since these people were born. Think how much more sugar and processed food we are eating, how many more chemicals we are exposed to, and how each generation has declined. We are now experiencing an epidemic of problems that were rare in earlier generations. People with food and chemical intolerance used to spend most of their lives at levels I and II stimulus. In old age, they would lose weight and begin getting neuropsychiatric conditions such as Alzheimer's disease. Now many people are getting mental symptoms while they are still young. They are thin, not because they are at level I stimulus, but because they are at level III withdrawal.

The following list of diseases and conditions that may involve a dysfunctional stomach is based on three criteria:

1. High levels of homocysteine are often present. High homocysteine usually stems from low levels of folate and B12. Low B12 levels are caused by hypochlorhydria (low stomach acid). High homocysteine is being used as a marker for poor stomach function.

2. On the withdrawal side, many more women than men have the condition. On the stimulus side, more men than women have the condition.

3. Within the last 50 years, there has been a major increase in the condition. It now seems as though there is an epidemic.

Withdrawal Conditions (primarily women)
- Migraines
- Asthma (adult women)
- Celiac disease
- Osteoarthritis
- EI, environmental illness
- MCS, multiple chemical sensitivity
- Vegetarianism (many, but not all, vegetarians)
- Chronic Fatigue Syndrome
- Fibromyalgia
- Anxiety disorders
- Depression
- Anorexia
- OCD, obsessive-compulsive disorder (equal numbers of men/women)
- Autoimmune diseases
- Alzheimer's disease

Stimulus Conditions (primarily men/boys)

- Asthma (boys as children)
- ADHD, attention deficit, hyperactivity disorder
- Alcoholism
- Tourette's syndrome
- Bipolar disorder (equal numbers of men/women)
- Autism
- Psychopathic personality
- Schizophrenia
- Parkinson's disease

Investigating each of these conditions in terms of allergies, B12, and homocysteine can provide clues. For example, anorexia has always been rather mysterious and inexplicable. How can a person who is emaciated refuse to eat because she is "too fat?" Earlier in this book, we discussed some of the mental symptoms of anorexia, which occur at level III withdrawal. Feelings of anxiety, self-loathing, and shame appear to be psychological. In reality, they stem from reactions to foods and chemicals. Let's combine these mental reactions with well-known B12 symptoms. These include loss of appetite, epigastric pain (poor digestion, full or bloated feeling after eating small or normal sized meals), and congestive heart failure.[271] Those with anorexia are also known to have high levels of homocysteine. It all fits. The allergies, the

B12 deficiency, and the high homocysteine levels all come from poor stomach function. How often are women with anorexia tested for adequate hydrochloric acid?

Lanugo is the name for the soft, downy, fine white hair that grows mainly on the arms and chests of female anorexics. It can also grow on the face, back, stomach, and other areas. It is usually found on anorexics suffering from severe weight loss and nearing starvation. It is often attributed to an effort of the body to trap heat and stay warm.[272] Could lanugo be a sign of a B12 deficiency? Could it be related to the fine hairs along the chin line many elderly women experience? We euphemistically call it "peach fuzz." When I started using B12 lozenges, my annoying peach fuzz started disappearing. I had had this problem for about 12 years so I couldn't expect it to disappear entirely, but it is about 60% better. Fine hair along the chin line may serve as a warning that older women need to check their vitamin B12 status. Lanugo may serve as confirmation that a B12 deficiency is involved in anorexia.

The title of this chapter is "Recovery." How are we ever going to recover our personal health, the health of our children, and the health of our nation? It all seems so impossible. If I am correct, and we are able to unravel the underlying causes of many degenerative health conditions, perhaps it will not be so impossible.

First, let's look at some factors that have enabled one modern nation to maintain high health standards. Japan is known to have the healthiest population of any large industrialized nation.

1. Sugar consumption is very low in Japan. In 1980, it was less than 50 pounds per person per year. That was equivalent to the sugar consumption in the United States and the United Kingdom a century earlier.[273]

2. In Japan, the lowest acceptable serum B12 level is 500 pg/ml.[274] The corresponding number in the United States is 200 pg/ml. In the United States, many people with B12 deficiency symptoms test in the gray area between 200 and 500 pg/ml and are told that their B12 levels are normal.

3. Japanese women have the highest intake of iodine of women anywhere in the world because of the seaweed they eat. They consume 100 times the United States RDA of iodine. Japanese women have the lowest incidence of breast cancer in the world, and the men have ten times less prostate cancer than men in the United States.[275]

Certainly we could lower our consumption of sugar. That is reduce sugar and not eliminate sugar. Iodine and B12 could be taken care of with changes in testing protocols and supplementation. A few simple changes could make a surprising difference in our national health picture. According to Guy Abraham, M.D., "Ortho-iodo-supplementation (when the body is saturated with sufficient iodine to supply all the tissues) may be the safest, simplest, most effective, and least expensive way to solve the healthcare crisis crippling our nation."[276]

Americans used to get ample amounts of iodine in their diet because iodine was used in bread and other bakery products as a dough conditioner and anti-caking agent. One slice of bread provided the daily RDA for iodine. Because of an unwarranted concern over people getting too much iodine from bakery products, iodine was replaced with bromine in the 1980s. Now we know this was a terrible mistake. Bromine is a toxic element that interferes with the absorption of iodine. The National Health and Nutrition Survey found iodine levels had declined 50% in the United States from 1971 to the year 2000.[277]

When searching for the causes of neuropsychiatric illnesses, inadequate levels of iodine must be considered along with homocysteine, B12 deficiency, allergies, and food intolerance. According to Dr. Brownstein, "Iodine deficiency sets up the immune system to malfunction." It may be involved in such conditions as fibromyalgia, chronic fatigue syndrome, and autoimmune disorders.[278] Adequate levels of iodine also help to detoxify the body through the increased urinary excretion of lead, cadmium, arsenic, aluminum, and mercury.[279]

Most people think they are getting enough iodine if they use iodized salt. However, this is not an adequate source of iodine. According to Dr. Abraham, "only ten percent of the iodine in iodized salt is absorbed. On a molar basis, there is 30,000 times more chloride than iodine in iodized salt. Chloride competes with iodide for absorption in the intestinal tract." [280] James Howenstine, M.D. writes that it is not feasible to correct an iodine deficiency by using iodized salt. It would require 20 teaspoons of iodized salt daily to get enough iodine.[281] For more information, read *Iodine: Why You Need It, Why You Can't Live Without It* by David Brownstein, M.D. To understand the latest research and the controversies surrounding iodine go to www.optimox.com and click on "research." Before changing your supplement program, work with your doctor and have him monitor your thyroid function. Some people are very iodine sensitive.

The consequences of a lack of either B12 or iodine during pregnancy or while breast-feeding can be severe. In utero iodine deficiency has been associated with many problems in children, which includes depression, cretinism, dwarfism, mental retardation, and even ADHD.[282] A lack of B12 has been associated with developmental delay, autistic-like symptoms, motor problems, loss of language and social skills, or failure to thrive. Many couples are unable to conceive due to a deficiency of these nutrients.[283] Dr. Brownstein's book on iodine and *Could It Be B12?* contain excellent information on the need for iodine and vitamin B12 during pregnancy.

Now we come to the most difficult part. What can we do about allergies? Avoiding everything we are reacting to and diagnosing our allergies and food intolerance isn't good enough. Avoiding all of our favorite foods leads to endless frustration. Allergies are one more degenerative health problem, which was unknown to those on traditional diets. This means that allergies do not have to be part of the human condition. What causes food intolerance and allergies? How can we prevent it?

Dr. Randolph showed us that hidden or "masked" allergies to common foods cause chronic health problems. If a person breaks out in a rash after eating a rarely eaten food, such as dates, he just doesn't eat dates again. But what if a child gets a slight stomach upset from eating a piece of bread? He will probably continue eating toast, cookies, cereal, and other products that contain wheat every day. In the early stages, he may get a lift or stimulus for several hours after he has wheat, but he needs more wheat every few hours to stay on this high. If he goes too long without a cookie or cracker, he will feel "all gone" or let down. He learns subconsciously that he needs some kind of a bread product to stay on his high and cookies and crackers become his favorite foods. Without realizing it, he has developed a wheat addiction. His parents usually don't realize he has a hidden allergy because he may seem very bright or just be a little overactive at level I stimulus. However, this chronic addiction to a food he is reacting to could lead to possible arthritis, migraines, or depression later in life. This type of masked allergy could develop from any commonly eaten food, such as milk, corn, eggs, or soy.[284]

We can no longer ignore allergies and food intolerance or tell patients that it is all in their head. Too many people know better. The key to understanding this whole area of medicine is the work of Theron Randolph, M.D. Dr. Doris Rapp dedicated her book, *Our Toxic World: A Wake Up Call*, to her patients and to Dr. Randolph:

> Theron Randolph, M.D. in the 1940s recognized chemical sensitivities and no one listened in spite of all his publications, books, and successes with patients when others had failed. He led the way but unfortunately was so far ahead of his times that he (was) not only unappreciated, but he was persecuted and ridiculed, much like Semmelweis. Bless him for all he taught to so many about this illness...[285]

This book has attempted to demonstrate the long-term consequences of our transition from traditional foods to the modern diet of Western civilization. This has been the great human experiment of the last 150 years. Our change in diet explains much about the degenerative diseases that have overtaken us and the cultural decay we see around us. We have studied:

1. The changes in personality and the deterioration in character

2. The degenerative diseases caused by our over consumption of sugar and the increase in insulin

3. The epidemic of neuropsychiatric diseases brought on by poor stomach function, which allows allergies, food intolerance, and B12 deficiency to increase

4. How Alzheimer's disease develops, how it can be prevented or postponed, and how caregivers can help Alzheimer's patients

With knowledge comes power. Look at your own life and think how you could improve your health and perhaps even your personality. Think how you could help a friend or family member. Now that you know more about some of the underlying causes, look at the world and its problems with new insight and perspective.

IN MEMORIAM

JANET DAUBLE
1942 – 2011

JANET DAUBLE, THE FOUNDER AND DIRECTOR of Share, Care, and Prayer, will be greatly missed. Through her personal relationships, prayers, and newsletter, she built a virtual sanctuary and a loving, caring place for those with environmental illness (EI), multiple chemical sensitivity (MCS), and other chronic health problems. Many with these health problems feel isolated and alone. Some may live in a trailer in the desert. Others rarely leave a chemically safe room in their house. Still others feel isolated by a lack of empathy from those dear to them. There were over 4,000 members at the time of Janet's passing. Share, Care, and Prayer wasn't just another website. It was a community, and Janet held it together with her love, talent, work, and prayers.

In the early 1980s, Janet visited me in Jacumba, California. She knew about me because I was making and selling reading boxes for those who are sensitive to the chemicals in ink and paper. We drove around the Jacumba, Boulevard, Campo area. This is a high desert area along the Mexican border with clean, dry air. Mountains to the west block pollution from San Diego and Los Angeles. We were both dreaming of buying land and starting a sanctuary for those with environmental illness. Instead, I returned to teaching, took care of my mother, and later started writing this book. Janet began a small, local support group for those with chronic illnesses in Arcadia, California. Later, she moved to Frazier Park, California, started Share, Care, and Prayer, and took care of her father.

Another person who was important to the Share, Care, and Prayer community is Carolyn Gorman. Carolyn has been the health educator for all the patients at the Environmental Health Center of Dallas for over 27 years. She provided the EI Answer Line. Carolyn is continuing the answer line to answer health or EI questions. Her number is (972) 964-8333. Her book, *Less Toxic Alternatives* (10th edition), is available on Amazon or through the American Environmental Health Foundation.

In June of 2008, I wrote Janet and asked permission to include her letter to the editor of the *Townsend Letter for Doctors and Patients* at the end of my book. It is a powerful letter that really gives people an idea of what it is like to suffer from environmental illness. Her letter granting permission read in part:

I am happy that you are writing a book. You were on the ground floor of the EI network and in providing special products that were so needed and scarce. So, you are well acquainted with everything related to EI. I agree with you that Alzheimer's patients can be helped. I will be glad to help you with information in any way I can.

As you read the following letter to the editor of the *Townsend Newsletter** and come to the true cause of Janet's serious health problems, keep in mind something I found in the *Share, Care, and Prayer Newsletter*, Vol. 26, 2009. Janet mentions that the doctor who correctly diagnosed all of her symptoms as food allergy also gave her a "long series of B12 shots."

Patients with a Myriad of Strange Symptoms Are Not Crazy or Stressed Out—Just Allergic

Editor:

I had never been a particularly strong or healthy child. After I learned to swim, I began having chronic ear and upper respiratory infections for which I took sulfa and penicillin. Before the vogue of ear tubes, my ear drum was punctured a few times; then I had X-ray treatment(s) on my Eustachian tubes. Later I had a polyp removed

* Reprinted with permission

from that same ear and, later yet, a mastoidectomy. But I am getting ahead of my story.

Even though I was often sick and never felt good, I had many interests and kept busy. I first became alarmed that I might have serious health problems when my natural athletic ability began to fluctuate and degenerate in my late teens. For example: the first time I water-skied, I came right up out of the water, and I quit skiing only when I got tired. The second time, I even practiced dropping one ski. But the third time was embarrassingly painful— embarrassing because I couldn't even get up on two skis, and the falls were very painful. The fourth time a friend said he would take time and work with me. He thought I was probably trying too hard. He was very patient; however, I could not do anything right, and I had to quit when I injured myself in one of my super-duper falls.

It was also alarming that I began having a problem with pain. I had always enjoyed playing volleyball and I had a good serve. But I had to give up playing when just hitting the ball or serving one time would cause my hands and wrists to hurt for hours. I found it excruciatingly painful to try to do exercises in my body mechanics class while sitting on the floor, or to lean my head back on the sink to have my hair washed at the beauty salon.

As I continued to add more and more symptoms to my repertory as the years went by, I felt very fortunate to be able to put myself through college by working full time at the student health center because medical care was convenient and free. My chart became very thick, but none of the medicines helped me—most made me worse. I vividly remember that the Antivert I took for vertigo made me so dizzy I almost passed out. At the age of 21 I was referred to an arthritis specialist after a slightly positive blood test for rheumatoid arthritis. After his exam, I was advised "if you have as much pain as you say you have, you should go to a psychiatrist."

Soon after seeing the arthritis specialist I had mastoid surgery and then a tonsillectomy for chronic sore throats. My ear did stop draining, but I had much more dizziness, and my sore/dry, sometimes throbbing, throat (which often cultured out to be strep) continued for another ten years.

In my late twenties I had new carpeting installed in my apartment. It smelled terrible. I could even taste it. And I could not sleep in my apartment for the first few nights. My chronic bronchitis, which started after my tonsils were removed, turned into viral pneumonia with green and yellow sputum. About that time I had an exterminator come after my use of Raid failed to stop the ants.

Over the years, the extreme connective tissue/ muscle pain, poor balance/coordination and other MCS symptoms, cognitive problems, extreme fatigue, problems with digestion (constipation, vomiting, hemorrhoids, loose intestinal wall, nausea), hormones (dysmenorrhea and PMS, eyes tearing, broken blood vessels, blurred vision, pain) and skin (cysts, adult acne, boils, seborrheic dermatitis, warts, athlete's foot, sties, cold sores, fever blisters, hangnails, itching, creepy crawly feelings), and infections (bladder, vaginal, throat, bronchial, upper respiratory) increased. My use of antibiotics increased as well, until I had an allergic reaction to Tetracycline, which affected my liver and I ended up in bed for about a month.

It was always a challenge to get up in the morning (had to roll out rather than sit up because of pain and weakness) following nights of little sleep. I slept with a pillow between my knees because of pain, I often woke up during the night with hand and feet numbness and back spasms, and I had to walk the floor with leg cramps. I also experienced terrible nightmares, and sleep-walking and talking. My bladder incontinence was always more of a problem at night as well. Then there were the nights I had to get up to vomit, and the mornings when I would wake up with the room spinning after having gone out to dinner the night before. I always just blamed this on bad food.

It became painful to hold a washcloth in the shower and to wash dishes, to stand long enough to wash dishes, to walk up and down stairs, and an occasional torticollis (neck spasm) did me in for several days. As my sense of smell increased, my sense of hearing decreased (except that my own chewing of food became very loud, and I thought everyone could hear me chew).

In my early thirties, I advanced to experiencing "psychological" symptoms. I began washing my hands a lot and was compulsive about checking and rechecking whether the stove and iron were off and the door locked. I now realize that the OCD was caused by my short-term memory loss. I also began to lose my keys or lock them inside the car or apartment, and I let my car run out of gas quite often. I developed some depression, irritability, and even paranoia for a short time. I could not concentrate long enough to read and understand one paragraph in the Bible or to pray.

It became increasingly difficult for me to type because of poor coordination and cognitive function, and I came to a point where I did not see how I could work any longer. (As I share this story, I wonder how I worked as long as I did!) I continued to see specialists, and search for a diagnosis in the *Merck Manual*, but since this was before environmental illness (EI), chronic fatigue syndrome, and fibromyalgia were being diagnosed, I had no basis for seeking disability status and had no other support.

With the advent of the "psychological" symptoms, I finally gave in and went to see a psychiatrist at the age of 34. How fortunate I was that he believed my symptoms were physical. He sent me to a specialist who "majored in puzzles." But, when baffled by my normal blood test and contradictory 24 hour urine tests, the specialist suggested having sex as the solution. (One chronically ill woman I know who was a wife, mother, and grandmother had been advised by a physician to have sex twice a day! She was correctly diagnosed as food and chemical sensitive later.) After I explained my belief about abstinence for singles, besides my fatigue and total lack of interest (my desire had also fluctuated to extremes over the years), he countered with, " If you would get your crooked tooth fixed, you might feel better about yourself." I had never even given my crooked front tooth a thought, and I had a high regard for myself, especially for being able to keep going under the circumstances of my health problems. So much for the puzzle-solver.

Through counseling and prayer with my pastor, I found out about hypoglycemia and found a doctor who treated it. In a five-minute visit, I told her that I was a "complete physical and mental basket case and had had about every test there was." She asked me if I had any allergies. I remembered that milk made my face break out and some perfume gave me a rash just where it was applied. She decided I needed to take one more test: a RAST test.

The test showed I was highly allergic to foods I was eating every day. I was surprised because I had never had hay fever or the usual allergy symptoms, and no foods seemed to bother me (except for the time I got hives from eating too many apricots as a child). And who would have believed that food allergy could have caused all the problems I had? Later, intradermal testing showed I was also somewhat allergic to hydrocarbons.

It was wonderful to know there was a reason for my degenerating health, and that I could get better. And, as time went by, I could look back on my life and clearly see why my health was better or worse depending on my diet and environment. I now knew why the five-hour glucose tolerance test just about killed me and made me sick for days. The doctor said the test results were not significant—but the drink was concentrated corn syrup, and I was highly allergic to corn! And since most medication contains corn in some form, it made sense that medicine, including my pain killers, made me sicker.

It was also a revelation to learn people are commonly addicted to the very foods that make them sick. As I read more food labels and became more knowledgeable, I realized that not only was I most attracted to Mexican food, but that just about every other food I enjoyed contained corn. For example, my morning fruit was canned in corn syrup. The brand of canned stewed tomatoes and spinach I liked contained dextrose. My favorite lunch restaurant made their fries in corn oil and their bread contained corn flour.

It was hard, but I did change my diet. And, once I stopped poisoning myself, I did get better! I no longer had chronic flus and colds, other infections, sleep and nerve problems during the night, sciatic nerve pain, or pains I thought might be heart attack, stroke, or appendicitis. My jaw stopped clicking, I didn't bite my tongue or lips anymore, and I didn't even need my glasses for the astigmatism. As my vocabulary and other cognitive skills increased, my depression, phobias, and compulsions decreased. At church I could sit through the sermon without my rear end going numb, I could cross my legs without them going numb or asleep, I could rise and sing right away instead of having to wait to have breath (usually by the third verse), I could close my eyes in prayer while standing up and not lose my balance, and my left arm no longer trembled while holding the hymnal. And it was with great joy, after years of not having balance or coordination or strength, breath or energy, that within six months of being on a strict diet, I was able to take up ice skating!

My health improved dramatically. When I was first diagnosed, I thought I was the only one with these crazy symptoms and severe food sensitivities. Then I began to help other chronically ill people. I started a local support group in 1983. This turned into a nonprofit organization in 1987, and the organization serves nearly 4,000 people today.

I so enjoy helping other people overcome their particular myriad of symptoms. My deepest regret, however, is not being able to reach people who have been diagnosed with chronic fatigue syndrome and fibromyalgia with the truth about this cause of chronic illness. I am grateful I found out about my food and chemical sensitivity before there were such established CFS and FM networks because, like these people, I might not have listened to the doctor when she suggested I have just one more test—*a food allergy test.*

There has been some recent progress made in the CFS network. Dr. Paul Cheney, a CFS expert, is now recommending food elimination diets. "The more I get into the issue of diet and food sensitivities, it's obvious to me that the single most common antigen to which we are exposed is food proteins. Elimination diets, and improving digestion and gut epithelial function can pay huge dividends...I've seen people in 30 days have huge clinical responses simply by this very simplest of moves." On his website, Dr. Cheney cites a German study, which found that 88% of those CRS patients studied had Type IV food hypersensitivity.

I recommend provocative/neutralization or machine testing by an environmental physician; RAST and ELISA/ ACT (by Serammune Physicians Laboratory) blood tests for immediate and delayed food sensitivities; keeping a diet/environment diary; and/or using an elimination or 4-day rotation diet.

It has been 22 years since I took the RAST test. It is hard always to be on a diet, and I would rather be able to take a pill. But I have my life back. I work full time at a stressful job, and on my days off I take care of my 90-year old father who lives 80 miles away. And, as I discovered, if allergens are not avoided, then the chronic illness is progressive, resulting in an increase of more and more debilitating and painful symptoms.

It is my prayer that researchers will study how toxic chemicals can cause a person to become sensitive and then find out how to rebalance the body. I am sure that it can be done. Current study into just pain or just fatigue is not broad enough, because chronically ill, sensitive patients react individually. One person who has become sensitive to wheat will have overwhelming fatigue and another, cognitive problems and another, pain.

Janet Dauble
Founder and Director
Share, Care, and Prayer, Inc.
January, 2001

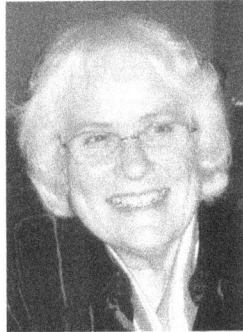

ABOUT THE AUTHOR

MARY ALICE BONWELL TAUGHT SPECIAL education in San Leandro, California when her health suddenly collapsed. Diagnosed with environmental illness and too sick to continue teaching, she went to live with her mother and started a small business selling reading boxes to those sensitive to chemicals in paper and print. Her reading boxes led her to medical conferences and enabled her to talk with hundreds of chemically sensitive patients. During this time, she learned the importance that Theron Randolph, M.D. and his research have to the whole field of environmental medicine. By following the precepts of Dr. Randolph, she largely regained her health and returned to teaching special education in Imperial, California.

While she was teaching, Mary Alice continued her professional studies and cared for her mother who had slipped into Alzheimer's disease. As she worked on writing her master's thesis, she talked with the director of the

Photo courtesy of Paul Soltow Jr.

Price-Pottenger Nutrition Foundation and utilized their materials. Weston Price, D.D.S. wrote about our physical degeneration over the period of several generations, but as MaryAlice worked with children affected by learning disabilities and coped with her mother's Alzheimer's, she began to realize that people could be degenerating mentally and emotionally as well.

Mary Alice graduated and received honors by the University of Washington's political science department. Mary Alice has been studying and writing on the political and cultural implications of a society that is degenerating both mentally and physically gradually over the span of several generations. In doing so, she continues to bring a unique perspective to the question of why our country is in decline.

BIBLIOGRAPHY

Abraham, G. E., J. D. Flechas, and J. C. Hakala.
"Orthoiodosupplementation: Iodine Sufficiency of the
Whole Human Body." Optimox Research Information.
2002. Accessed 19 Nov. 2011. www.optimox.com.

"Allergy and Environmental Illness." Woodlands Healing Research
Center. 9 Feb. 2007. Accessed 9 Nov. 2010. www.woodmed.
com/allergy.htm.

"Alzheimer's Disease: The Baby boomer's Nightmare." Accessed 8
Oct. 2010. www.csmngt.com/alzheimer.htm.

Bader, Walter. *Toxic Bedrooms: Your Guide to a Safe Night's Sleep.*
IL: Freedom Publishing Company, 2007.

Baines, Surinder, Jennifer Powers, and Wendy J. Brown. "How
does the health and wellbeing of young Australian
vegetarian and semi-vegetarian women compare with
non-vegetarians?" *Public Health Nutrition.* 13 Feb. 2006.
Accessed 16 Oct. 2010. www.journals.cambridge.org.

Bauerlein, Mark. *The Dumbest Generation.* New York: Jeremy P.
Tarcher/Penguuin, 2008.

Bock, Kenneth, and Cameron Stauth. *Healing the New Childhood
Epidemics: Autism, ADHD, Asthma, and Allergies.* New
York: Ballentine Books, 2007.

Boyd, D. B. "Insulin and cancer." *PubMed.* 2 Dec. 2003. Accessed 20
Jun. 2012. www.ncbi.nim.nih.gov/pubmed/14713323.

Braly, James and Patrick Holford. *The H Factor Solution.* North
Bergen, NJ: Basic Health Publications, Inc. 2003.

Brostoff, Jonathan and Linda Gamlin. *Food Allergies and Food Intolerance*. Rochester, VT: Healing Arts Press, 2000.

Brownstein, David. *"Clinical Experience with Inorganic Non-radioactive Iodine/Iodide."* 2005. Accessed 19 Nov. 2011. www.optimox.com.

———*Iodine: Why You Need It, Why You Can't Live Without It*. West Bloomfield, MI: Medical Alternatives Press, 2009.

Bruno, Anthony. "If You Look At Me Again, I'll Shoot You." *Crime Library*. Accessed 17 April 2007. ww.trutv.com/library/crime/serial_killers/.../ramirez/arrest_5.html.

"Bulimia: symptoms, causes, treatment, complications, long-term outlook." Accessed 7 Jun. 2010. www.mamashealth.com/bulimia.asp.

"Cancer Facts." Reproduced from American Cancer Society. Accessed 29 Jun. 2012. www.thomlatimercares.org/Cancer_Facts.htm.

Christy, Martha M. *Your Own Perfect Medicine*. Scottsdale, AZ: Future Med, Inc., 1994.

Cleave, T. L. *Peptic Ulcer*. Bristol: John Wright & Sons LTD, 1962.

Conley, Mikaela. "Robots to Help Children With Autism" *ABC News*. 20 Oct. 2011. Accessed 11 May 2012. www.abcnews.go.com>Health.

Cowan, Thomas. "Gastroparesis." *Weston A. Price Foundation*. 27 Sep. 2004. Accessed 19 May 2012. www.westonaprice.org/ask-the-doctor/gastropareses.

De Silva, Padmal and Stanley Rochman. *Obsessive-Compulsive Disorder: The Facts* (3rd edition). New York, NY: Oxford University Press, 2004.

Diamond, John. *Your Body Doesn't Lie.* New York, NY: Warner Books, 1979.

"Dietary Supplement Fact Sheet: Vitamin B12." 24 Jun. 2011. Accessed 8 Feb. 2011. www.ods.od.nih.gov/factsheets/ vitaminb12-HealthProfessional.

Doheny, Dathleen. "Belly Fat in Midlife, Dementia Later?" *WebMD Health News.* 26 Mar. 2008. Accessed 15 Aug. 2011. www. webmd.com/

Dommisse, John V. "This book accurately chronicles the devastation caused by B12 deficiency." Amazon book review for *Could It Be B12?* 7 Sep. 2006. Accessed 18 Jun. 2012. www.amazon.com/Could-It-Be-B12.

Eades, Michael R. and Mary Dan Eades, *Protein Power.* New York: Bantam Books, 1996.

————— *The Protein Power Life Plan.* New York NY: Wellness Central, 2001.

————— "Tough meat for vegetarians to swallow." 18 Apr. 2006. www. proteinpower.com/drmike/archives/2006/.

Fallon, Sally and Mary Enig. *Nourishing Traditions.* Washington: New Trends Publishing, 2001.

"Fibromyalgia." *Immuno Laboratories. Inc,* Accessed 1 Dec. 2011. www.betterhealthusa.com/public/222cfm.

Fife, Bruce. *Stop Alzheimer's Now.* Colorado Springs, CO: 2011.

"Fluorescent Lights: The Danger Overhead." *Inform.* 13 Aug. 2004. Accessed 8 Jul. 2007. www.informic.org.

Friedman, Meyer and Ray H. Rosenman. *Type A. Behavior and Your Heart.* New York: Fawcett Crest, 1974.

"The friendly robot for autistic kids." *The Week.* 10 Mar. 2011. Accessed 11 May 2012. http://theweek.com.

Galst, Liz. "Global Worrying: "The environment is in peril and anxiety disorders are on the rise. What's the connection?" *Plenty* magazine, August/September 2006. Accessed 8 Aug. 2012. www.plentymag.com/magazine/global_worrying.php.

Gedgaudas, Nora T. *Primal Body, Primal Mind.* Rochester, VT: Healing Arts Press, 2011.

Goleman, Daniel. *Social Intelligence.* New York: Bantam Dell, 2006.

Gorman, Carolyn, and Marie Hyde. *Less-Toxic Alternatives (Ninth Edition).* Optimum Publishing, 2004.

Grandin, Temple. *Thinking in Pictures.* New York: Vintage Books, 1995.

Grohol, John M. "Statistics: Europeans Have Mental Health Issues Too." Psych Central World of Psychology. Accessed 5 Sep 2012. Psychcentral.com/.../statics-europeans-have-mental-health-issues-to…

Hale, Julianne. "Understanding Anorexia Nervosa." *Chattanooga HealthScope.* Summer 2008. Accessed 23 Jul. 2012. www.healthscopemag.com.

Hancock, David. "Should Malvo's Confession Be Tossed?" *CBS News*. 11 Feb 2009. Accessed 14 Sep 2012. www.cbsnews. com

Harley, Willard F. "Why Women Leave Men." *Marriage Builders*. (Reprinted and edited from *New Man Magazine* 1995-2012). Accessed 3 Apr. 2007. www.marriagebuilders.com.

"Helicobacter Pylori." *Medicine Net*. Accessed 28 Apr. 2010. www. medicicenet.com.

Heylighen, F. "Increasing Intelligence: the Flyn Effect." *Principia Cybernetica Web*. 22 Aug. 2000. Accessed 12 Apr. 2012. http://pespmcl.vub.ac.be/FLYNNEFF.html.

Hoffman, Ronald. "Alzheimer's disease." www.drhoffman.com/ page...cfm/89.

Howenstine, James. "Iodine Is Vital For Good Health." *News With Views*. 5 Nov. 2005. Accessed 18 Nov. 2011. www. newswithviews.com.

"In Her Own Words: Living With Anorexia and Bulimia." *Lifescript.* Accessed 23 Jul. 2012. www.lifescript.com.

Jackson, Mark. *Allergy: The History of a Modern Malady*. London, UK: Reaktion Books, 2006.

Johnson, DK, CH. Wilkins, and JC. Morris. "Accelerated weight loss may precede diagnosis in Alzheimer disease." Washington University School of Medicine, St Louis, MO. Sep. 2006. Accessed 20 Aug. 2011. PubMed [PMID: 16966511].

"Kaspar the friendly robot teaches autistic children how to enjoy a simple hug." *Daily Mail*. 9 Mar. 2011. Accessed 11 May 2012. http://www.dailymail.co.uk.

Keith, Lierre. *The Vegetarian Myth.* Crescent City, CA: Flashpoint Press, 2009.

Krajocovicova-Kudlackoya, M, et al. "Homocysteine levels in vegetarians versus omnivores." *PubMed.* 2000. Accessed 17 May 2010. www.ncbi.nih.gov/pubmed/11053901.

Kupelian, David. "Almost 40 percent of Europeans are 'mentally ill." *Whistle Blower.* December 2011: 7.

Kushi, Michio. *Your Face Never Lies.* London: Red Moon Press, 1976.

Larson, C, et al. "Lifestyle-related characteristics of young low-meat consumers and omnivores in Sweden and Norway." *Journal of Adolescent Health.* 2009. Accessed 17 Oct. 2010. www.lycos.com/info/vegetarianism--meat.html.

Lee, Dennis. "How is *H. pylori* infection diagnosed?" *Medicine Net.* Accessed 16 Jun. 2012. www.medicinenet.com/helicobacter_pylori/page3.htm.

Lindeman, Marjaana. "The state of mind of vegetarians: Psychological well-being or distress?" University of Helsinki, Finland. 2002. Accessed 17 Oct. 2010.

Luchsinger, J.A. and D.R. Gustafson. "Adiposity and Alzheimer's disease. Current Opinion in Clinical Nutrition & Metabolic Care." Jan. 2009. *Pub Med* [PMID: 19057182].

Mallaby, Sebastian. *More Money than God. CSPAN After Words.* FT 5 Sep. 2010.

Mandell, Marshall and Lynne Waller Scanlon. *Dr. Mandell's 5 Day Allergy Relief System.* New York: Thomas Y. Crowell Publishers, 1979.

Mackarness, Richard. *Eating Dangerously*. New York: Harcourt Brace Jovanovich, 1976.

—— *Living Safely in a Polluted World*. New York: Stein & Day. 1983.

—— *Not All In the Mind*. London: Pan Books Ltd, 1976.

McGee, Charles T. *How to Survive Modern Technology*. Alamo, CA: Ecology Press, 1979.

Morrisey, Beth. "Lanugo and Eating Disorders." *Eating Disorder Expert*. 23 Dec. 2010. Accessed 26 May 2012. http://www. eatingdisorderexpert.co.uk.

Murray, Charles. *Coming Apart*. New York: Crown Forum, 2012.

Natenshon, Abigail. "Becoming Vegetarian? Be Sure to Become a 'Smart' One." *Empowered Parents*. Accessed 3 Nov. 2010. www.empoweredparents.com.

Newport, Mary T. *Alzheimer's Disease: What If There Was a Cure?* Laguna Beach, CA: Basic Health Publication, Inc., 2011.

Nohlgren, Stephen. "Spring Hill couple's Alzheimer's fight tries boost in brain superfuel." *St. Petersburg Times*. 3 Aug. 2009. Accessed 25 Mar 2010. www.tamabay.com/news/health/ research/article1924137.ece.

Norman, Eric J. "How May Thousands Be Prevented from Developing Alzheimer's Disease?" Norman Clinical Laboratory, Inc. 20 Feb. 2008. Accessed 18 Aug. 2011. www. b12.com/.

"On Growing Old with Environmental Illness: An Interview with Theron G. Randolph" *The Human Ecologist*. Fall 1991: 13-15.

Owens, Robbie. "Arlington Developers Hope Their Robot Helps Autistic Kids." *CBSlocal*. 26 Apr. 2012. Accessed 11 May 2012. http://dfw.cbslocal.com.

Pacholok, Sally M. and Jeffrey J. Stuart. *Could It Be B12?* Fresno, CA: Quill Driver Books, 2011.

Page, Melvin E. and Leon Abrams, "Cave-man and Primitive Peoples—What Lessons Do They Teach Us?" (Excerpts from *Your Body Is Your Best Doctor*). *Health & Healing Wisdom: The Price-Pottenger Nutrition Foundation Journal*. Fall 2007: 14-16.

Papolos, Demitri F. and Janice Papolos. *The Bipolar Child*. New York: Broadway Books, 1999.

Penn, Mark J. and E. Kinney Zalesne. *Microtrends*. New York: Twelve, 2009.

Pierini, Carolyn. "Eliminating the Surprising Culprit Behind Stomach Concerns." *Vitamin Research News*. January 2010: 1, 4, 5.

Pottenger, Francis Marion. *Pottenger's Cats: A Study in Nutrition*. Lemon Grove, CA: Price Pottenger Nutrition Foundation, 1995.

Price, Weston A. *Nutrition and Physical Degeneration*. (50th Anniversary Edition). New Canaan CT: Keats Publishing, Inc., 1989.

"Protein Nitration Influences Allergic Reactions." *FWF Austrian Science Fundpress* release. Accessed 15 Jun. 2012. www.fwf.ac.at/en/public_relations/press/pv201004-2en.html.

Randolph, Theron G. and Ralph W. Moss. *An Alternative Approach to Allergies (Revised Edition)*. New York: Harper & Row, Publishers, 1980, 1989.

—— *A Bibliography: 60 Years of Published Works*. 1997.

—— *Environmental Medicine: Beginnings and Bibliographies of Clinical Ecology*. Clilnical Ecology Publications, Inc., 1987.

Rapp, Doris J. *Is This Your Child?* New York: William Morrow and Company, Inc., 1991.

—— *Is This Your Child's World?* New York: Bantam Books, 1996.

—— *Our Toxic World: A Wake Up Call*. Buffalo, NY: Environmental Medical Research Foundation, 2004.

—— *Recognize and Manage Your Allergies*. New Canaan, CT: Keats Publishing, Inc., 1987.

Raymond, Eric S. *New Hacker's Dictionary* (3rd edition). Cambridge MA: MIT Press, 1998.

Rea, William J. *Chemical Sensitivity, Volume 1: Principles and Mechanisms*. Boca Raton, FL: Lewis Publishers, 1992.

—— *Chemical Sensitivity, Volume 3: Clinical Manifestations of Pollutant Overload*. Boca Raton, FL: Lewis Publisher, 1996.

Reisberg, Barry. "Seven Stages of Alzheimer's." *Alzheimer's Association*. Accessed 11 Sep. 2011. www.alz.org/alzheimers_disease_stages_of_alzheimers.asp.

Rogers, Joseph. "High-Sensitivity C-Reactive Protein: An Early Marker of Alzheimer's?" *Journal Watch/Annals of Neurology*. 11 Oct. 2002. Accessed 12 Oct. 2011. www.neurologyjwatch.org.

Rogers, Sherry A. *No More Heartburn*. New York: Kensington Books, 2000.

Rowen, Robert Jay. "Symptoms of Iodine Deficiency." *Second Opinion Newsletter*. October, November 2004. Accessed 15 Dec. 2011. Quoted at www.trueknowledge.com/q/iodine_deficiency_symptoms.

"The Safe and Effective Implementation of Ortho-iodo-supplementation in Medical Practice." *Iodine Medical Conference*. 4-6 Oct. 2007: Coronado, CA. Accessed 10 Sep. 2011. www.fibromyalgiarecovery.com/IODINE.

Schechter, Harold. *The Serial Killer Files*. New York: Ballantine Books, 2003.

Schmidt, Reinhold, et al. "Early inflammation and dementia: A 25-year follow-up of the Honolulu-Asia aging study." *PubMed*. 2002. Accessed 9 Sep. 2011. www.ncbi.nim.nih.gov/pubmed/12210786.

Shallenberger, Frank. "The Complete Cancer Treatment Plan." Real Cures Healing Series, Volume 2. 2009: 1-8.

——— "How to Knock Out Digestive Problems Once and For All." *Real Cures Healing Series, Volume 2*. 2009: 39-44.

——— "How to Reverse Alzheimer's Disease." *Real Cures Healing Series, Volume 1*. 2011: 48-53.

Silberstein, Susan. "Unraveling the 'Type C' Connection: Is There a Cancer Personality?" *Healing Cancer*. Accessed 6 Jul. 2012. www.healingcancer.info/book/export/html/37.

Smart, Joanne McAllister. "The gender gap: if you're a vegetarian, odds are you're a woman." *Vegetarian Times*. Feb. 1995.

Accessed 16 Oct. 2010. www.findarticles.com/p/articles/mi-m0820/is.../ai-16019829/.

"Smarter than ever." *The Week.* 16 Sep. 2011: 11.

Snowdon, David. *Aging with Grace.* New York: Bantam Books, 2002.

————— "Brain infarction and the clinical expression of Alzheimer's disease: The Nun Study." *Nun Study Publication Abstracts.* 16 Dec. 2008. Accessed 15 Aug. 2011. www.nunstudy.org.

Stanger, Olaf, et al. "Homocysteine, folate and vitamin B12 in neuropsychiatric diseases: review and treatment recommendations." *Expert Reviews Neuother.* 2009: 1393. Accessed 10 Dec. 2011. www.expert-reviews.com.

"Statistics on Bulimia." *Bulimia Help.* 3 Mar. 2010. Accessed 7 Jun. 2010. www.bulimiahelp.org.

Stein, Rob. "Study Links Middle-Age Belly Fat to Dementia." *Washington Post.* 27 Mar. 2008. Accessed 12 Aug. 2011 www.washingtonpost.com.

"Supplements helpful for fibromyalgia." *Supplement News.* Accessed 2 Dec. 2011. www.supplementnews.org/wiki/fibromyalgia.

Taubes, Gary. *Good Calories, Bad Calories.* New York: Anchor books, 2007.

————— "Is Sugar Toxic?" *New York Times Magazine.* 13 Apr. 2011. Accessed 5 Nov. 2011. www.nytimes.com2011/04/17magazine/mag-17sugar-t.html.

————— *Why We Get Fat.* New York: Alfred A Knopf, 2011.

Untersmayr, E. and E Jensen-Jarolim. "The effect of gastric digestion on food allergy." *Current Opinion Allergy and Clinical Immunology*. 6 Jun. 2006: 214-219. [PubMed ID: 16670517].

Untersmayr, Eva, et al. "Antacid medication inhibits digestion of dietary proteins and causes food allergy." *The Journal of Allergy and Clinical Immunology*. September 2003: 616-623.

———— "The effects of gastric digestion on codfish allergenicity." *The Journal of Allergy and Clinical Immunology*. February 2005: 377-382.

"Veganism in a Nutshell." *The Vegetarian Resource Group*. Accessed 20 Jul. 2012. www.vrg.org.

"Vitamin B12 for Fibromyalgia & Chronic Fatigue Syndrome." *About.com*. 28 Oct. 2010. Accessed 2 Dec. 2011. www.chronicfatigueabout.com.

Wagner, Aureen Pinto. *What to do whenYour Child has Obsessive-Compulsive Disorder*. Lighthouse Press, Inc., 2006.

Whitmer, RA., et al. "Central obesity and increased risk of dementia more than three decades later." *Neurology Journal*. 26 Mar. 2008. Accessed 12 Aug. 2011. www.neurology.org/lookup/...01.wn10000306313.89165.efv1?...

———— "Obesity in middle age and future risk of dementia." *BMJ (British Medical Journal)*. 11 Jun. 2005, Accessed 20 Aug. 2011. PubMed Central.

Williams, David. "Prevention Is Easier Than Hoping for a Cure." *Alternatives Newsletter*. January 2012: 3.

———— "Just When You Think You've Heard It All, Urine for Another Surprise." *Alternatives* Vol. 5, No. 14. August 1994.

Wright, Jonathan V., and Lane Lenard. *Why Stomach Acid Is Good for You*. Lanham, MD: M. Evans, 2001.

———— "No more wheezing! Uncover the surprise cause of your grandchild's asthma." *Nutrition & Healing Newsletter.* December 2010: 1-7.

———— "Thinning hair and chipped nails: The serious health threat lurking behind these so-called 'cosmetic' conditions." *Nutrition & Healing Newsletter.* April 2010: 1-3.

Zabriskie, Nieske. "Helicobacter Pylori's Destructive Role: From Alzheimer's to Heart Disease and Beyond." *Vitamin Research News.* April 2010: 6, 7.

Zaciragic, A., et al "Elevated serum C-reactive protein concentration in Bosnian patients with probable Alzheimer's disease." *J Alzheimer's Dis*. 12 Sep. 2007. Accessed 15 Oct. 2011. www.ncbi.nim.nih.gov/pubmed/17917159.

Zaki, Jamil. "What, Me Care? *Scientific American Mind*. January/February 2011: 14, 15.

ENDNOTES

1	Grohol.
2	Williams, "Prevention Is Easier Than Hoping for a Cure." p. 3.
3	Taubes, *Good Calories, Bad Calories*, p. 92.
4	"Smarter Than Ever," p. 11.
5	Zaki, p. 15.
6	Grohol.
7	Price, pp. 23-25.
8	Price, p. 26.
9	Price, p. 37.
10	Price, p. 38.
11	Price, p. 40.
12	Price, pp. 42, 43.
13	Price, p. 44.
14	Price, p. 48.
15	Price, p. 49.
16	Price, p. 46.
17	Price, pp. 56, 57.
18	Price, p. 57.
19	Price, pp. 91, 131.
20	Price, pp. xv, xvi.
21	Pottenger, pp. 6-10.
22	Pottenger, pp. 10-12.
23	Pottenger 10, 11.
24	Conversation with Pat Connolly, former director of the Price-Pottenger Nutrition Foundation.
25	Pottenger, pp. 2, 6.
26	Pottenger, pp. 22-25, 31.
27	Pottenger, p. 33.
28	Mandell, p. 8.
29	Pottenger, p. 35.
30	Jackson, pp. 58-69.
31	Mackarness, *Living Safely in a Polluted World*, pp. 41, 42.
32	Mackarness, pp. 41, 42.
33	Mackarness, p. 11.
34	Mackarness, *Not All in the Mind*, pp. 57-61.

35   Randolph, *Environmental Medicine,* pp. 96, 97.
36   Mackarness, p. 60.
37   Mackarness, p. 63.
38   Randolph, p. 24.
39   Randolph, *An alternative Approach to Allergies,* pp. 16-19.
40   Randolph, pp. 40-48.
41   Randolph, pp. 41-43.
42   Randolph, pp. 41, 42, 44, 45, 129.
43   Randolph, pp. 41, 45, 46.
44   Randolph, pp. 41, 46.
45   Randolph, pp. 41, 42, 47.
46   Randolph, pp. 41, 42, 47.
47   Randolph, pp. 41, 48.
48   Randolph, pp. 41, 48.
49   Randolph, pp. 202+
50   Grandin, pp. 59, 66.
51   Papolos, p. 14.
52   Hancock.
53   Harley.
54   Raymond.
55   Raymond.
56   Raymond.
57   Rapp, *Is This Your Child's World?,* pp. 79-114.
58   Schechter, pp. 103, 104.
59   Bruno.
60   Bock, p. 38.
61   Grandin, pp. 15, 87-89.
62   Friedman, pp. 86-106.
63   Grandin, p. 44.
64   Grandin, p. 96.
65   "Veganism in a Nutshell."
66   Keith, p. 62.
67   Fluorescent Lights: The Danger Overhead."
68   Galst, p. 1.
69   Mallaby.
70   Raymond, p. 527.
71   Price, p. 27.
72   Friedman, p. 226.
73   Friedman, pp. 110, 111.
74   Goleman, p. 7.
75   Conley.

76   "The friendly robot for autistic kids."
77   "Kaspar the friendly robot teaches autistic children how to enjoy a simple hug."
78   ABC News, p. 2.
79   Owens.
80   Randolph, pp. 139-147.
81   Hale.
82   "In Her Own Words: Living With Anorexia and Bulimia"
83   *Obsessive-Compulsive Disorder*, pp. 1-69, 37.
84   Wagner, pp. 34-35.
85   De Silva, p. 19.
86   De Silva, p. 67.
87   De Silva, pp. 25 – 27.
88   Rapp, *Is This Your Child's World?*, pp. 107,108.
89   Rapp, p. 109.
90   Rapp, p. 91.
91   Rapp, p. 107.
92   Rapp, p. 72, 75.
93   Rapp, p. 81.
94   Rapp, *Is This Your Child?*, pp. 142, 423.
95   Rapp, *Is This Your Child's World?*, p. 102.
96   Rapp *Is This Your Child?*, p. 369.
97   Rapp
98   Silberstein, p. 1.
99   Silberstein, pp. 2, 3.
100   Silberstein, p. 3.
101   Randolph, *An Alternative Approach to Allergies,* pp. 153, 171.
102   Rapp, *Is This Your Child's World?*, p. 21.
103   Friedman, pp. 112, 113, 118.
104   Friedman, pp. 107-112.
105   Friedman, pp. 113-118.
106   Randolph, *An Alternative Approach to Allergies,* pp. 47-48.
107   Galst, p. 2.
108   "Smarter than ever," p. 11.
109   Heylighen, p. 1.
110   Heylighen, p. 2.
111   Murray, p. 43.
112   Wright, "Thinning hair and chipped nails."
113   Kushi, p. 31.
114   Untersmayr, "The effect of gastric digestion on food allergy."

115   "Protein Nitration Influences Allergic Reactions." p. 1.
116   Untersmayr, "The effects of gastric digestion on codfish
        allergenicity."
117   Wright, *Why Stomach Acid Is Good for you*, pp. 28-29.
118   "Protein Nitration Influences Allergic Reactions," p. 1.
119   Untersmayr. "Antacid medication inhibits digestion
        of dietary proteins and causes food allergy."
120   Untersmayr. "Antacid medication inhibits digestion."
121   Untersmayr. "The effects of gastric digestion on codfish
        allergenicity."
122   Untersmayr. "The effect of gastric digestion on food allergy."
123   Untersmayr. "The effects of gastric digestion on codfish
        allergenicity."
124   Wright. *Why Stomach Acid Is Good for You*, pp. 113,114.
125   Rea. *Chemical Sensitivity, Volume 3*, p. 1431.
126   Shallenberger, Vol. 2, p.42.
127   Roger, pp. 90-91.
128   Pacholok, p. 222.
129   "Dietary Supplement Fact Sheet: Vitamin B12."
130   Braly, p. 119.
131   Eades, "Tough meat for vegetarians to swallow."
132   Pierini, p. 5.
133   Wright. *Why Stomach Acid Is Good for You*, pp. 22, 130.
134   Shallenber, *Real Cures Healing Series*, Vol. 2, p. 41.
135   Wright. "Thinning hair and chipped nails," pp. 2, 3.
136   Wright, p. 3.
137   Wright, p. 3.
138   Lee, pp. 1-2.
139   Rogers, p. 151
140   Shallenberger, Vol. 2, p. 43.
141   Gedgaudas, p. 56.
142   Wright, *Why Stomach Acid Is Good for You*, p. 152.
143   Shallenberger, Vol. 2, p. 43.
144   Wright, p. 147.
145   Rea, pp. 262,263.
146   "Allergy and Environmental Illness," p. 8.
147   Browstoff, pp. 6, 7.
148   McGee, pp. 138, 147.
149   Browstoff, p. 119.
150   Browstoff, p. 34.
151   Mcgee, p. 138.

152	Browstoff, p. 35.
153	Gedgaudas, pp. 41, 42, 274.
154	Rapp, *Is This Your Child's World*, pp. 82, 405.
155	Diamond, pp. 32, 60, 61.
156	Rapp, p. 53.
157	Rapp, pp. 21-22.
158	Randolph, *An Alternative Approach to Allergies*, p. 206.
159	Randolph, p. 47.
160	McGee, p. 146.
161	Rapp, *Is This Your Child?*, p. 171.
162	Rea, *Chemical Sensitivity, Vol. 3*, p. 1431.
163	Rapp, p. 171.
164	"Bulimia: symptoms, causes, treatment, complications, long-term outlook."
165	Rapp, *Recognize and Manage Your Allergies*, pp. 14.
166	Braly, pp. 69, 70.
167	"Alzheimer's Disease: The Baby Boomer's Nightmare."
168	Randolph, *An Alternative Approach to Allergies*, pp. 28, 139.
169	Penn, pp. 187, 188.
170	Bains.
171	Larson.
172	Lindeman.
173	Natenshon.
174	Keith, p. 230.
175	Keith, p. 193.
176	Keith, p. 234.
177	Eades, *The Protein Power LifePlan*, pp. 3-8.
178	Eades, p. 9.
179	Eades, *Protein Power*, p.9.
180	Page, p. 15.
181	Taubes, *Good Calories, Bad Calories*, pp. 25-26.
182	Eades, *The Protein Power LifePlan*, p. 26.
183	Eades, *Protein Power*, p.11.
184	Eades, pp. 299, 300.
185	Boyd.
186	Shallenberger, "The Complete Cancer Treatment Plan," p. 5.
187	McGee p. 152.
188	Rea, pp. 368-370.
189	Fallon, p. 112.
190	Taubes, "Good Calories, Bad Calories," pp. 145-151.
191	Gedgaudas, p. 139-161.

192   "On Growing Old with Environmental Illness," pp. 13-15.
193   Williams, "Just When You Think You've Heard It All Urine for Another Surprise."
194   Christy.
195   Pacholok, pp. 18-21, 39.
196   Snowdon, *Aging with Grace*, pp. 52-61.
197   Snowdon, pp. 48, 93.
198   Snowdon, pp. 89-91.
199   Snowdon, pp. 79, 215.
200   Snowdon, pp. 86, 95.
201   Snowdon, pp. 155, 156.
202   Snowdon, p. 179.
203   Eades, "Tough meat for vegetarians to swallow."
204   "Dietary Supplement Fact Sheet: Vitamin B12," p. 5.
205   Snowdon, "Brain infarction and the clinical expression of Alzheimer's disease."
206   Norman.
207   Zabriskie, pp. 6, 7.
208   Cowan, p. 1.
209   Snowdon, pp. 91-92.
210   Rogers.
211   Whitmer.
212   Johnson.
213   Luchsinger.
214   Pacholok, p. 39.
215   Snowdon, p. 155.
216   Reisberg, p. 4.
217   Pacholok, p. 18-20.
218   Pacholok, p. 24.
219   Wright, p. 145.
220   Pacholok, p. 41.
221   Hoffman.
222   Hoffman.
223   Hoffman.
224   Hoffman.
225   Hoffman.
226   Hoffman.
227   Dommisse.
228   Brownstein, p. 91.
229   Gorman.
230   Nohlgren.

231   Newport, pp. 55-61.
232   Newport, pp. 57-68.
233   Newport, pp. 141, 157, 158.
234   Newport, pp. 265, 266.
235   Shallenberger, Vol. 1, pp. 48-53.
236   Newport, p. 240.
237   Newport, p. 227.
238   Taubes, p. 90.
239   Taubes, pp. 92-93.
240   Taubes, p. 93.
241   Taubes, p. 93.
242   "Cancer Facts," p. 2.
243   Taubes, p. 116.
244   Eades, *Protein Power*, p. 10.
245   Taubes, p. 91.
246   Taubes, p. 454.
247   Taubes, "Is Sugar Toxic?"
248   Taubes.
249   Taubes, *Why We Get Fat*, p. 188.
250   Taubes, *Good Calories, Bad Calories*.
251   Eades, pp. 316-318.
252   Taubes, pp. 212-218.
253   Taubes, pp. 222-223.
254   Taubes, p. 136.
255   Taubes, pp. 137-138.
256   Taubes, *Why We Get Fat*, p. 112-126.
257   Gedgaudas, p. 139.
258   Cowan.
259   Stanger, p. 1393.
260   Kupelian, p. 7.
261   Kupelian, p. 7.
262   Williams, "Prevention Is Easier Than Hoping for a Cure,"
       p. 3.
263   Papolos, p. 25.
264   Cleave, p. 31.
265   Cleave, p. 79.
266   Abraham.
267   Rowen.
268   Brownstein, *Iodine: Why You Need It, Why You Can't Live
       Without It*, pp. 89-90.

269   Randolph, *An Alternative Approach to Allergies,* p. 26.
270   "On Growing Old with Environmental Illness: An Interview with Theron G. Randolph," p. 14.
271   Pacholok, p. 19.
272   Morrisey.
273   Taubes, p. 117.
274   Norman.
275   Howenstine.
276   Abraham.
277   Brownstein, *Iodine: Why You Need It, Why You Can't Live Without It,* p. 40.
278   Brownstein, "Clinical Experience with Inorganic Non-radioactive Iodine/Iodide."
279   Abraham.
280   Abraham.
281   Howenstine.
282   Brownstein, *Iodine: Why You Need It, Why You Can't Live Without It,* p. 196.
283   Patcholok, pp. 177, 213.
284   Randolph, pp. 26-27.
285   Rapp, *Our Toxic World.*

PROFESSIONAL CREDITS

This book would not have been possible without the help of talented professionals in the publishing industry. The author would especially like to thank the following people:

Ellen Reid	Ellen Reid's Book Shepherding
Robert Henry	Book Editor
Deborah Perdue	Illumination Graphics
Pamela Guerrieri	Proofed to Perfection
Clive Pyne	Clive Pyne Book Indexing Services

INDEX

Thinking in Pictures and Other Reports from My Life with Autism (Grandin), 49, 65
tight joints, 177
tooth decay, 4, 7–10
Tourette's syndrome, 277
The Toxic Bedroom (Bader), 180
traditional diet. *See also* diets
cancer, does not cause, 267
cancer absent with, 1
cod's head stuffed with chopped cod's liver and oatmeal, 10
food preservation by drying, salting, and fermenting, 13
immunity to disease, high, 12
of isolated Swiss, 6–7
oatcake and oatmeal porridge, fish organs and eggs, 11–12
organic and locally grown, unsprayed produce, 187
processed foods diet vs, 5, 7–9
raw meat, 13
raw milk, 138
seafood, domesticated animals, game, dairy products and a variety of fruits, vegetables, grains, and legumes, 13
stamina and superb physiques, 10–11
strength and stamina of people, 10, 12
tuberculosis and modern diet vs., 8, 10
whole rye bread, cheese, and raw milk from goats or cows, 6, 9
triglycerides, 254, 266, 268
Type A Behavior and Your Heart (Friedman and Rosenman), 68, 82
Type A personality, 94. *See also* attention
acquaintances, hundreds of, 83
feeling of being overstressed, 68
food and chemical intolerance, 68
food intolerance, 40–41

hypersensitive immune system, 68
level I stimulus, 41, 68
level II stimulus, 42, 68
overstimulated personality, 68
Type C personality ("C" is for cancer), 114–17
emotional repression; unassertive; unaware of anger feelings; self-sacrificing; prone to guilt and self-blame, 114
level III withdrawal, 108, 116–17, 127
poor memory, 117
type I diabetes, 258
type II diabetes, 200

U
UBT. *See* urea breath test (UBT)
ulcerative colitis, 24
ulcers
bulimia and, 185
cabbage juice and healing of, 158
H. pylori and, 150, 272
mastic gum and, 159
Native Americans and, 263
NSAIDs and, 159
refined carbohydrates and, 272
stomach lining inflammation and, 150
traditional diets and, 272
United States
Alzheimer's or senile dementia, 187
cancer and, 1
cancer deaths, 263
feelings of depression, guilt, anxiety, and helplessness, 1
heart attacks, 187
iodine levels, 273, 280
IQ scores in, 127–28
neuropsychiatric disorders, 270–71
prostate cancer, 279
sense of community, lack of, 138
sugar consumption, 264, 279

– 347 –

www.ingramcontent.com/pod-product-compliance
Lightning Source LLC
Chambersburg PA
CBHW062155270326
41930CB00009B/1546